Personalized Diet and Fitness

Leonard B. Walz

Acknowledgements

Whatever you do, give your best and you will never have regrets.

This project is dedicated to my family. Several of my family members have suffered from food allergies and chronic conditions such as type 1 diabetes, type 2 diabetes, high blood pressure, diverticulitis, gluten intolerance, nut allergy, and egg sensitivity. My family has struggled for years to find recipes that everyone can eat and enjoy, especially during Holiday meals. This concept was inspired by my mother's dedication to cooking and the countless hours she spent researching and creating new recipes that everyone could eat. This project was designed with my family's experiences in mind. Hopefully this project can help more families easily create meals they can all enjoy together adhering to each family member's dietary restrictions, all while saving time.

Thank you to my family, friends, mentors, CSUB faculty, and Alumni Association who have supported me along the way and have believed in my dreams. Thanks to their support, I am the first in my family to receive a master's degree.

I am filled with gratitude to all the organizations who supported my lifelong dream and have awarded me with scholarships throughout my educational journey. Thank you to Mrs. Haas who assisted me with applying to the master's program and to Mrs. Rogers who supported me with career development support and an internship opportunity. You have both inspired me to become a mentor for the youth and assist them in finding their dream careers.

A special thanks to Professor Woods who has served as my committee member for my thesis and has guided me throughout my educational journey.

Thanks to Dr. Moore, Professor Commuri, Mr. Hernandez, and Mrs. Hernandez who advised me in counseling and made it possible for me to graduate in a year. Thank you for believing in my capabilities and allowing me to participate in the Fast Track Program. Thank you to Professor Frampton, Professor Woods, Professor Arias, and Professor Xu who provided me with the educational background to make me a successful graduate student. Thank you to Professor Sohail and Professor Norris who has provided me with a great education on APA formatting and teaching me project management concepts.

A special thanks to my brother who always made sure I was safe during the night classes and my Dad who would always get me the study snacks. Nina, Yaya, Auntie Maryellen, and Auntie Kathy for always supporting my educational journey. Kat, who would always sit with me as I worked on my project, your support does not go unnoticed.

Thank you, Dr. Pallitto, for always willing to help me with my new ideas and providing me with feedback and guidance. I am thankful that you have given me the opportunity to try out my ideas. I am grateful to have worked with you and Dr. Martinez during the summer internship and I have gained experience working in a school office setting.

I am thankful to God for letting me discover my dream career at an early age and to make what once was a dream at an early age, a reality.

I am proud to say that I am now a locally homegrown double alumni of CSU Bakersfield. I am grateful for the education that I have received, and I am thankful that I was able to receive two high quality educations debt free, without having to leave my hometown. I am looking forward to my future career and I am confident that I am well prepared to face my next journey in life.

Abstract

Noncommunicable diseases have increased in the frequency found in patients in the United States' population. With a large shortage of healthcare resources, and a shortage of dietitians and nutritionists, these limited healthcare resources have produced long wait times to receive nutritional resources. The literature suggested that an intervention is needed to alleviate the dietitian shortage. The purpose of this research was to build a business proposal for a recipe generator app that will create recipes custom to each patient's health dietary restrictions. The study also addressed the research questions: a) What are the problems that need to be solved?, (A lack of healthcare resources and there is a nutritionist and dietitian shortage; noncommunicable diseases are on the rise; and patients lack time and education to research recipes.), b) How would a business proposal for the Build My Diet Health App be developed?, and c) Will the app be a profitable solution that will solve patients' needs? This study used a nonexperimental qualitative content analysis of the reviews from the Apple® App Store® that used a qualitative coding technique of secondary data to provide insight on user needs. This study used a two-step market research process and analyzed eighty – three textual sources. The first step was to a) conduct a competitor analysis; and the second step was to b) perform qualitative coding on app reviews to discover emerging themes of user's insights. Findings of the emerging themes are as follows: a) *easy to use, simple, easy features, integrates,* and *syncs,* b) *love app* and *great app,* c) *lose wight,* and d) *feel accomplished, achieve goals,* and *goals.* This study suggested the Build My Diet Healthcare App can be a successful and profitable business idea.

Table of Contents

List of Figures

Chapter 1 – Introduction and Background

The Jones family is gathering the ingredients for their traditional Thanksgiving family cooking party and are about to go shopping when they get a phone call from grandma. She says she was diagnosed with diverticulitis and can no longer eat anything that has seeds. Auntie Barbara has type one diabetes, the nephew, Jeffy, has a gluten intolerance diet, and Phil has diabetes. The family wonders to themselves what can we all eat now? The family does not want to cook everyone separate dishes because it will be too much work, so the nephew pulls up the App Store® and finds an app that can generate Thanksgiving themed recipes that they can all eat. This is the perfect solution to their Thanksgiving problem.

Caring Hospice is expanding with their number of residents. Each resident has different multiple health diets, and it is becoming difficult for the staff to create new meals for their residents. The CEO has noticed that while the staff tries their best to follow each patients' diets, the family members of the patients have complained that some of the meals they are serving do not adhere to what they should be eating. The CEO is becoming frustrated with all the complaints and sees his staff is doing their best to comply with the diets, but it is hard to keep track of all of them. He thinks to himself there must be a better way. Afraid of a potential lawsuit and always wanting to give the best quality care possible, the CEO goes to the web to find a solution, when he finds a mobile health software application that will assist him with his problem. It is the perfect solution to his nightmare because the staff can enter in each patient by diet health constraint, input their likes and dislikes, can keep the staff organized, and can generate instant recipe ideas for each patient.

Anna is a young single mother who has two daughters and must find time to care for her two young children and work to provide for her family. Her older daughter has a peanut allergy, her younger daughter is lactose intolerant, and Anna is diabetic. Anna has tried researching recipes that everyone in her family can eat without having to cook separate meals, but this takes up too much time and each diet is complicated to learn. The girls are picky eaters and are getting tired of the recipes she creates. Anna is about to give up when she discovers a recipe generator app. This app is different from the other meal planning apps. This one just doesn't give you general recipes for a certain health condition diet, it allows you to choose all the diets you have and combine them into one recipe. Anna is skeptical at first, but she tries it and discovers that it also has a family section, so you can add multiple family members' diets and create one meal everyone can enjoy together. Anna is relieved to finally have found a solution and gone are the days of cooking everyone's separate meals! With the app, Anna and her girls have been able to adhere better to their diets and it has made it quicker and faster to create recipes.

All these composite stories have in common a shared problem, patients need an easier method to manage their chronic health conditions diets. Imagine you have been diagnosed with a health condition; the doctor gives you a suggested printout of what you cannot eat. You drive home, open the fridge, and think to yourself now what can I eat? With the mobile health software application that will be described in this research, it will turn a now what situation into you knowing exactly what you can make. My research is creating a business proposal for a mobile healthcare app that will help patients create custom recipes that combine their health condition's dietary restrictions all with one phone swipe. The proposed app has a unique feature of differentiation because the app creates custom recipes for each patient tailored to their personal health conditions, and patients will no longer spend countless hours researching recipes that adhere to all their diets. The Build My Diet Health App is focused on a niche to assist patients with their self-management of their dietary constraints caused by chronic conditions. Some potential competitors contain recipes for chronic conditions; but they do not combine several diets together to adhere to a patient's full need of combining all their dietary restrictions into one recipe. Patients will be more likely to stick to their diet with an app that can do the research for them of new recipes. The mobile health software application is created with different people's stories in mind. All of them are unique to their circumstances, but they share that they can benefit from the mobile health software application, as a solution to their needs.

Purpose of the Study

The purpose of this research project is to develop a business proposal for a recipe generator nutritional app that can create custom recipes that will adhere to the patient's custom health dietary restrictions such as allergies, chronic diseases, noncommunicable diseases or mental health diets. The purpose of this app is it will assist patients to create custom recipes that can adhere to their health diets and patients will have a more efficient, accessible, and timesaving way to adhere to their diets; and it can improve patient health outcomes and prevent health complications. Also, reducing risk factors for noncommunicable diseases could prevent almost 39 million deaths by 2030, such as implementing a healthy diet, not smoking, exercising regularly, moderating alcohol intake, and reducing exposure to air pollution (Harvard T.H. Chan School of Public Health, 2023). Developing a business proposal for the mobile health software application can help educate patients and provide them with customizable recipes that can suit their needs. This app can help patients eat healthier and adhere to their health diets by providing them with an accessible tool that will save their time and create custom recipes based on their diets needs.

Noncommunicable diseases

Noncommunicable diseases also known as, NCD's, are chronic diseases that are caused by unhealthy lifestyle patterns. Some noncommunicable diseases include cancer, diabetes, heart disease, and stroke. Noncommunicable diseases are preventable and creating health interventions can reduce the amount of people who suffer from these diseases. Noncommunicable diseases kill 41 million people each year, equivalent to 74% of all deaths globally. Each year, 17 million people die from a NCD before age 70. Cardiovascular diseases account for most NCD deaths, or 17.9 million people annually, followed by cancers, 9.3 million, chronic respiratory diseases, 4.1 million, and diabetes, 2.0 million including kidney disease deaths caused by diabetes (World Health Organization, 2022). The mobile health software application will focus on noncommunicable diseases since they are one of the main leading causes of death in the United States. The app will have a selection menu that the patient can choose the conditions they suffer from, and the app will generate recipes based on their diet health needs. The app will also have a food likes and dislikes section to not only customize it to what the user should be eating, but what they actually enjoy eating and it will adhere to all their diets. The literature research shows there is a need for the app and key statistics are summarized about the prevalence and impact of noncommunicable diseases on a nationwide level. Harvard's T.H. Chan School of Public Health (2023) pointed out some key facts about noncommunicable diseases in the U.S.

United States Noncommunicable Diseases Key Facts:

- 70% of annual deaths are due to chronic diseases.

- These preventable conditions compromise quality of life and add to the rising health care costs—75% of our health care dollars are devoted to treating these diseases. Diabetes is the leading cause of kidney failure, non – traumatic lower extremity amputations, and blindness amongst adults. Chronic diseases can be preventable by making diet and lifestyle changes to reduce your risk and prevent chronic diseases.

Problem and Severity

Noncommunicable diseases are occurring more often in society. People are suffering from several health conditions which impact their diets, such as chronic diseases, food allergies, and noncommunicable diseases, and they lack the knowledge and time to create recipes for their diet. By 2030, chronic diseases will account for 70% of total global deaths and 56% of the global disease burden, coupled with an estimated cumulative production deficit of $47 trillion between 2011 and 2030. This epidemiological change will also place tremendous pressure on the health systems of nations, especially those in the least developed countries, as they must be confronted with a double burden of acute and chronic diseases amidst scarce resources (Sabila, 2020). The literature shows there is an ever-growing problem with noncommunicable diseases; and interventions will need to be created to address these shortages of healthcare resources and lower healthcare costs. Also, every $1 invested in proven NCD interventions will generate at least $7 in increased economic development or reduced health care costs by 2030 (Davidson, 2020). The mobile health software application described in this thesis can serve as a possible solution to address these rising problems of cost and lack of resources. It is profitable for the healthcare industry to invest in mobile health app interventions to reduce healthcare costs and increase accessibility. Also, a growing number of aging adults, more prone to developing chronic diseases, such as heart disease and diabetes, drives demand for industry services. Nutritionists and dietitians help these aging adults stay active and involved by developing a special diet for them. The number of adults aged 50 and older is expected to increase in 2022 (IBIS, 2022). With an increase in population that has more than one chronic disease, a tool is needed to help dietitians create recipes that can assist patients and alleviate the dietitian shortage. There will be a national shortage of RDNs by 2020 and the field will experience 16 percent growth in job opportunities between 2014 and 2024 (Cooper, 2019). Mobile health apps can provide an accessible and low-cost intervention to assist patients and lead to better patient health diet adherence rates. Healthcare costs are rising along with the cost of noncommunicable diseases (Figure 1).

Figure 1

Ballooning Costs of Health Impacts in Food Systems

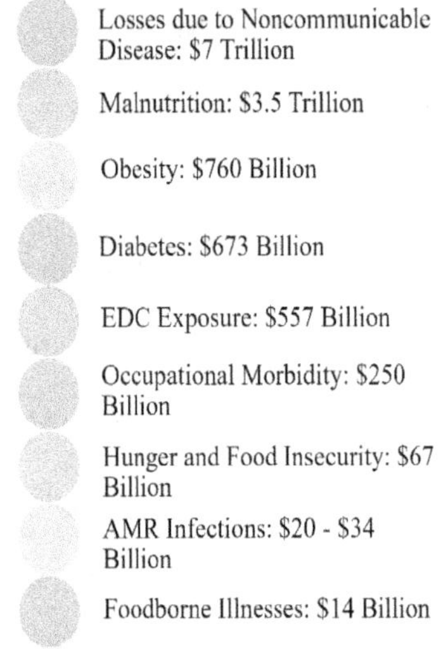

Note. Transforming the food system to fight non-communicable diseases, adapted from Branca, F., et al. (2019). *Transforming the food system to fight non-communicable diseases.* (https://doi.org/10.1136/bmj.l296).

Significance of the Study

Examining the literature, it was found the nutrition industry does have a large market size for growth and revenue. User penetration of the nutrition app industry will be 4.22% in 2023 and is expected to hit 4.96% by 2027 and the average revenue per user is expected to amount to US $15.29 (Statista, 2023). It is important to examine the market research reports on the related industries to see if it will be a feasible research project before creating a business proposal for a new mobile health software application. Since both market research reports show there is a need and potential for market size growth and revenue, it will be worthwhile to form a business proposal for the mobile health software application. Also, the increasing incidence of lifestyle diseases, growing concerns about inadequate nutrition, and a large geriatric population are some of the key factors responsible for the rising demand for retained nutrition products (Grand View Research, 2018). As patients see how having several health conditions can impact the quality of life, people are wanting more tools and preventive interventions to prevent health complications. Also, there are more mobile devices in the world than there are people. By 2026, mobile applications are projected to generate $233 billion in revenue (Velvetech, 2023). This shows there is a growing demand for nutritional support, and this suggests there is a large need for the mobile health software application described here.

The mobile health software application will be developed initially for the U.S. market. North America dominated the personalized nutrition and supplements market with a share of 41.51% in 2022. This is attributable to rising product awareness and increased spending on health and wellness across the U.S. and Canada (Grand View Research, 2018). Since the U.S. has one of the largest needs in the industry, the mobile health software application will be developed and marketed to users in the U.S. Please see Appendix C for more charts and figures of the market research of the nutrition app industry. A summarized illustration of the market report show the basic facts about nutrition and dietitian industry, the nutrition and supplements industry, and the mobile app industry (Figures 2, 3, and 4).

Figure 2

Personalized Nutrition And Supplements Market Report Scope

Report Attribute	Details
Market size value in 2023	USD 49.52 billion
Revenue forecast in 2030	USD 131.62 billion

Growth rate	CAGR of 15.0% from 2023 to 2030 to reach USD 131.62 billion by 2030.
Base year for estimation	2022
Historical data	2018 - 2021
Forecast period	2023 - 2030
Quantitative units	Revenue in USD million/billion and CAGR from 2023 to 2030
Report coverage	Revenue forecast, company ranking, competitive landscape, growth factors, and trends
Segments covered	Ingredient, dosage form, distribution channel, age group, region
Regional scope	North America; Europe; Asia Pacific; Latin America; MEA
Country scope	U.S.; Canada; Germany; U.K.; France; Italy; Spain; Denmark; Sweden; Norway; China; Japan; India; South Korea; Australia; Thailand; Brazil; Mexico, Argentina; South Africa; Saudi Arabia, UAE; Kuwait

Note. Personalized Nutrition And Supplements Market Report Scope, adapted from Grand View Research. (2018). *Personalized nutrition and supplements market size, share & trends analysis report by ingredient (vitamins, minerals), by dosage form (liquids, powders), by age group, by distribution channel, and segment forecasts, 2023 - 2030.* (https://www.grandviewresearch.com/industry-analysis/personalized-nutrition-supplements-market-report).

Figure 3

Global App Store® and Google Play® Spending 2021 - 2026

Revenue: $642.6 Million
Profit: $83.5 Million
Wages: $227.3 Million

Profit Margin: 13%
4,263 Businesses
5,913 Employment

Note. Global App Store® and Google Play® Spending 2021 - 2026, adapted from Velvetech. (2023). *Mobile app development process: Ultimate guide to build an app.* (https://www.velvetech.com/blog/mobile-app-development-process/).

Figure 4

Industry Report

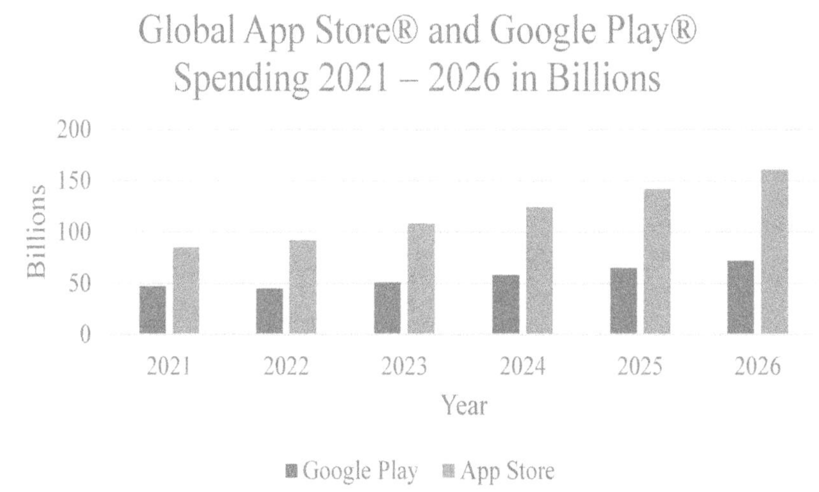

Note. Industry at a Glance, adapted from IBIS World. (2022). *Industry report OD5460: Nutritionists and dietitians in the U.S.* (https://my-ibisworld-com.falcon.lib.csub.edu/us/en/industry-specialized/od5460/about).

Methods

The methodology used for collecting sources included only sources from the Walter Stiern Library One Search, Google Scholar™, published textbooks, and credible website sources. For the Walter Stiern Library One Search and Google Scholar™, only peer reviewed sources and textbooks were included to use as sources. Although the textbooks are not peer-reviewed, they do go through a publishing process, and this makes it a credible source to use. The majority of the sources used are published in the year 2017 or newer. Older sources were only used if they were for explaining theories or foundational historical research. Website sources were only included if it was a credible source that has article reviewing procedures or comes from a standardized industry leader, such as the CDC or American Heart Association to name just a few. Credible website sources used include

.gov, .edu, .org, and only .coms that are unbiased established institutions that offer industry expertise and do not contain ads. Originally, three hundred and forty-nine sources were analyzed and read to see if it would be a useful, credible source that met the research criteria. In the end, eighty-three sources were used throughout the research paper. This research paper uses credible sources as the basis and foundation of the research to form a business proposal for the mobile health software application.

Chapter two literature review research will explain basic business theories such as the business proposal, strategic management framework, and app development steps guidelines. The business plan includes basic business theories such as a competitor analysis, SWOT analysis, and strategic management concepts just to name a few. The business plan and strategic management framework will serve as the main organizational framework of the research and will contain basic business planning concepts that are typically found in a business plan such as an executive summary, mission statement, and marketing plan just to name a few. The app development guideline was created using the industry recommended app development steps and examining case studies found in the literature with recommendations of successful app development. The purpose and main goal of this research is to develop a business proposal for a mobile health software application. The research does include a summarized overview of app development steps, but this is included only to give readers insight of the basic steps to develop an app to provide background and context before creating the business proposal in detail. The app development steps are not comprehensive because the main goal of the research is to develop a business proposal for the app. The organization structure used for chapter two is the inverted pyramid, also known as the funnel structure. This structure will start with a broad overview of the research topic, and it will narrow down the topics to the specifics of why the business plan is chosen. The theoretical framework shows the theories and concepts used throughout the research (Figure 5).

Figure 5

Theortical Framework: Inverted Pyramid (Funnel Structure)

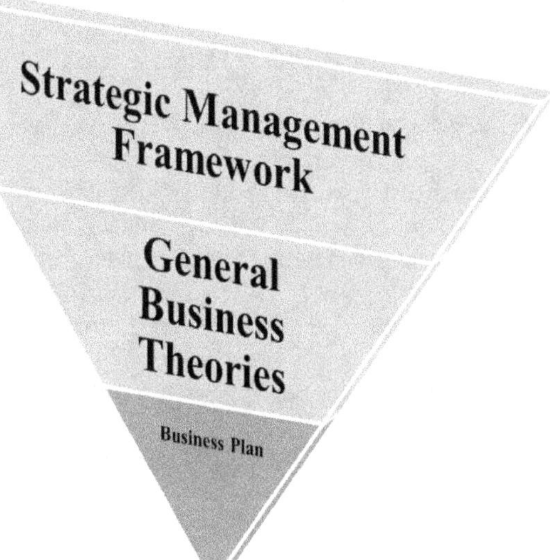

One of the methodologies that will be used includes using a qualitative content analysis to survey the Apple® App Store® market. This will compare the ratings and reviews of the main app competitors in the nutritional health app market and compare app rankings and features. As part of chapter three, a qualitative content analysis of the reviews from the Apple® App Store® will be included to analyze the market and competitors. This research will be beneficial to include because the app user reviews will provide further insight on user needs in a real-life setting. While the sources from the literature provides insight on need and overall industry problems, the qualitative content analysis of the reviews from the Apple® App Store® can give insights into the problems users are directly facing. Since the App Store® reviews are publicly available data, this does not contain privacy issues of data collection. As a method to further protect privacy of the app sore reviewers, the reviews will be deidentified to provide anonymity. This will include excluding any reviews that contain personal names and only including the review into the dataset. Since the username is not needed, the username will not be included in the dataset. The method to create the qualitative descriptive statistic will be to gather the data from the 2023 *top categories of health and fitness* and *medical app categories* from the Apple® App Store®. This will analyze the *top free, top paid,* and *best nutrition tracking app categories*. All these categories are related to the research topic at hand; and provide a thorough analysis of any potential competing apps. Then the data can be downloaded and transferred to Excel™ or SPSS - RStudio™ to analyze the data reviews in a qualitative setting. Then the reviewers will be de-identified by only including the review and organizing the reviews into thematic concepts. The data does not portray any particular organization or person in a subjectively bad light because it only uses factual, publicly available data that was made available to the public. This will provide credibility to the research because it reduces and mitigates against biases.

Chapter 2- Literature Review

This chapter will review the literature and provide the reader with a subject matter expert overview on the topics of business theories and concepts, mobile apps, diet constraints, and lack of healthcare resources, alongside a nutritionist shortage. I will use a patient centric focus approach by finding a solution to a problem that will focus on individual diet constraint needs and how the lack of healthcare resources and shortage of nutritionists can impact the nutrition industry landscape.

This research will have a focus on business background, alongside healthcare industry needs to form a viable solution to the patient's needs. I am proposing to create a mobile health software application that considers the need, that currently, there is not a solution to help ease the burden of diet adherence to noncommunicable diseases such as diabetes, heart disease, cancer, and stroke, just to name a few. The literature uncovers the need for developing technological solutions to address chronic diseases and assist patients in taking care of their health. The literature has uncovered there is not currently a solution that will help patients manage their care of multiple noncommunicable diseases. This app will assist patients in creating recipes custom to their personalized dietary needs and will consider that a one size fits all approach is not effective in nutrition. The databases used to search for the literature included sources from the Walter Stiern One Search, Google Scholar™, credible online sources, and published textbooks. Some example search terms used to find the sources include *non-communicable diseases, health apps, business model canvas, strategic management, and healthcare, Ansoff matrix, shortage of dietitians and nutritionists, app development, business proposal, recipes, diet guidelines,* and *diet prevent and diet adherence.*

Figure 6

The Systematic Review of the Search Process of the Literature Review Sources

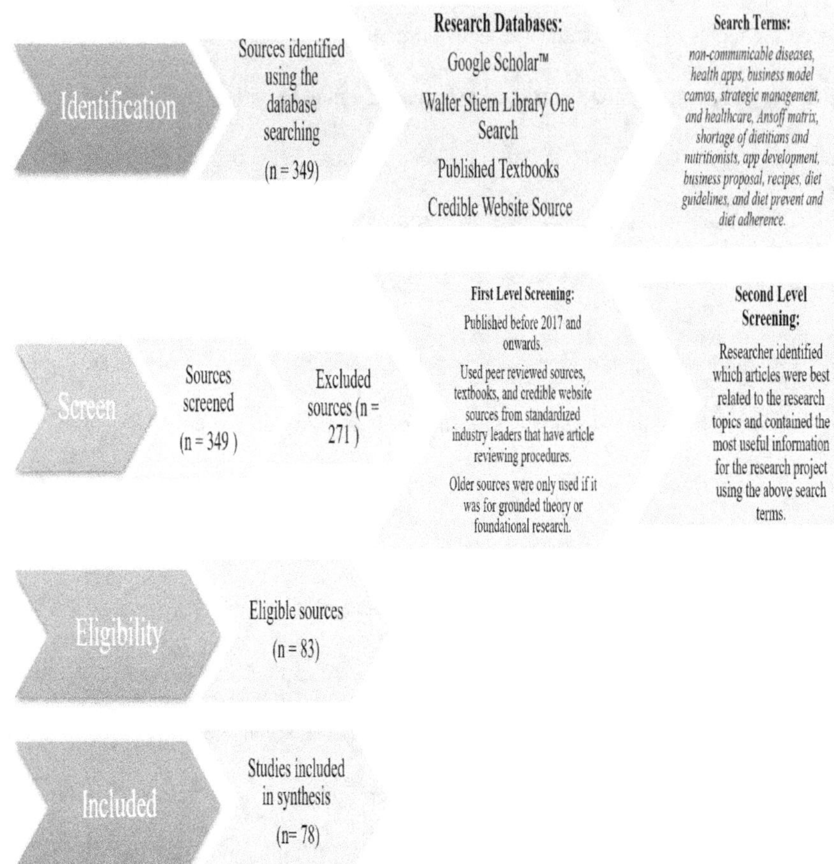

Before developing the business proposal for the mobile software application, it is imperative to look to the literature and research the basic topics that will impact the development of the business proposal such as diet constraints, the lack of healthcare resources, mobile apps, and business theories and concepts (Figure 6). This chapter will provide more background on these subjects to provide the reader with a well-researched understanding of the topics at hand (Figure 7).

Figure 7

Conceptual Model and Literature Map

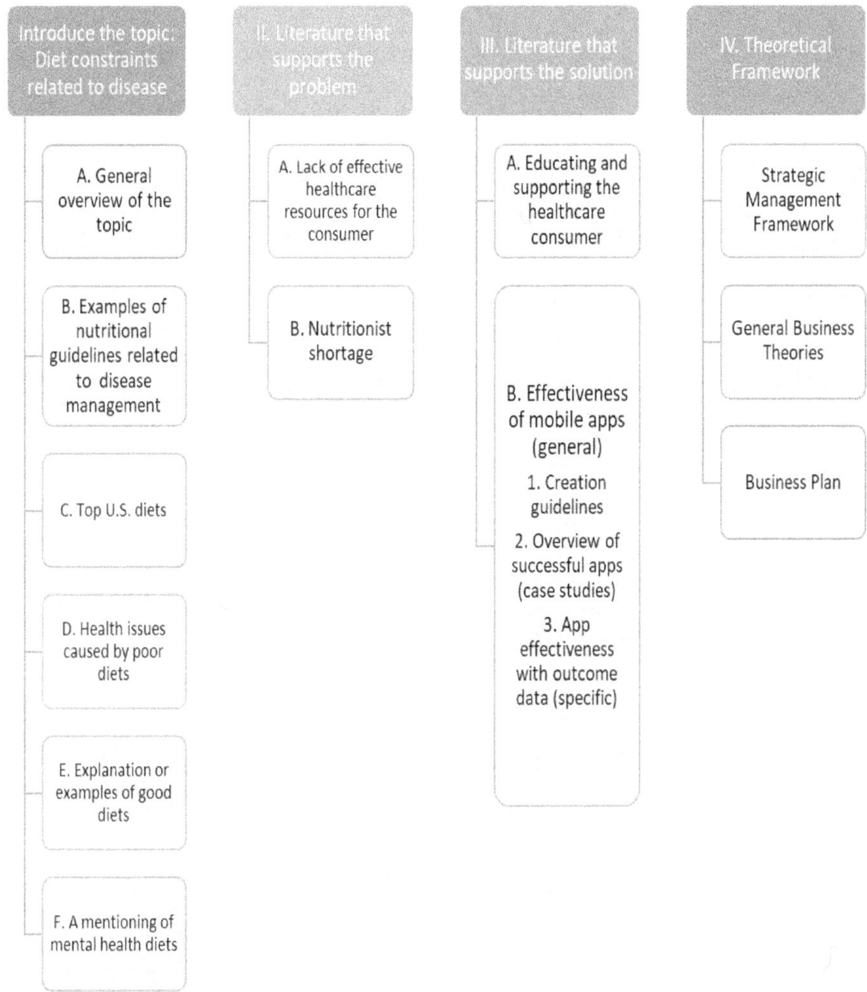

Diet Constraints Related to Disease

The mobile health software application bridges the gap of a lack of nutritional education and the

complex application of diet guidelines for chronic diseases the patient faces daily. For example,

evidence on the association between dietary patterns and reduced risk of diet-related chronic

diseases has expanded in recent years and supports the use of dietary patterns as a foundation for the recommendations in the Dietary Guidelines for Americans, 2020-2025. Consistent evidence demonstrates that a healthy dietary pattern is associated with beneficial outcomes for all-cause mortality, cardiovascular disease, overweight and obesity, type 2 diabetes, bone health, and certain types of cancer (U.S. Department of Agriculture & U.S. Department of Health and Human Services, 2020). Incorporating the USA dietary guidelines into the mobile health software application will assist patients in meeting their daily nutritional intakes. The diet adherence rates in the U.S. populations illustrate the healthy eating index scores (Figure 8).

Figure 8
Health Eating Index Scores

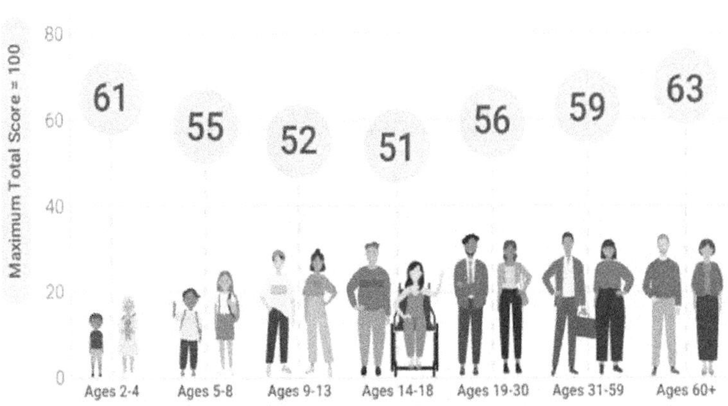

Note. Adherence of the U.S. Population to the Dietary Guidelines Across Life stages, as measured by average Total Healthy Eating Index Scores, by U.S. Department of Agriculture & U.S. Department of Health and Human Services. (2020). *Dietary guidelines for Americans, 2020-2025*. (https://www.dietaryguidelines.gov/sites/default/files/2020-12/Dietary_Guidelines_for_Americans_2020-2025.pdf). In the public domain.

Diet adherence is important for patients to adhere to because diet is related to nutrient deficiencies and following unhealthy diet patterns can cause noncommunicable diseases. Most American adults fail to meet daily recommendations for healthy behavior. Fewer than 18% of

American adults meet the daily recommendations for fruit and vegetable servings, only 10% of young adults entering college (18 to 30 years of age) are likely to adhere to dietary guidelines (Krzyzanowski et al., 2020). Adding an app feature into the mobile health software application will be beneficial to incorporate in the app. It can assist patients to reach their daily needed recommendations of fruit and vegetables to prevent malnutrition and noncommunicable diseases.

When patients research what they can eat for a health condition, there are recipes available based on one health condition, but there is a lack of recipes for patients that suffer from several chronic conditions. Also, food choices and food preferences of the person are important to their health. Even when a doctor prescribes a diet, a person has the right to choose foods that he/she likes. It is important that the person be included when planning menus and those food preferences of the person are taken into consideration when planning for doctor prescribed diets (TN Department of Intellectual and Developmental Disabilities, 2017). It is difficult for patients to educate themselves on all their diet guidelines, and then create their own recipes based on their diets. Also, many factors influence consumers 'dietary behaviors, from personal—such as culture, knowledge, skills, dietary preferences, and time for food preparation—to economic and political—such as the cost or availability of food. Information about food, whether education influences choices (Branca et al., 2019). This type of diet research is extremely time intensive for patients and it decreases their quality of life because they spend the majority of their time researching what they can eat. Patients get tired of eating the same foods and the mobile health software application can help introduce a new variety of recipes they can try based on their preferences. This section of research will cover research about nutrition guidelines and health issues fact sheets to show what each diet will include for noncommunicable diseases, food allergies, mental health diets, and the top U.S. health diets. The research will also cover sample menus and sample recipes to demonstrate the type of recipes that can be used for the mobile health software application. It is important to cover these topics because the nutritional guidelines and health fact sheets will serve as a foundation for the development of the mobile health software application.

Examples of Nutritional Guidelines Related to Disease Management

Analyzing the literature, fact sheets and nutritional guidelines are the most credible sources to obtain information about different health conditions diets because they were obtained from the Physicians Committee for Responsible Medicine. To provide a detailed and thorough analysis of the different types of diets for the different types of health conditions, I have included in my research nutritional guidelines and diet fact sheets. Please refer to appendix F to view all the health issues fact sheets and nutritional guidelines for noncommunicable and chronic diseases. It is important to research the basic health issues fact sheets and nutritional guidelines to understand each diet and to research what the diet includes to create accurate recipes for the mobile health software application. This can help in the future creation of the app because each fact sheet and guideline provide an understanding of all the different types of diets, and this will be used as one of the foundational aspects of the app.

Top U.S. Health Diets

A healthy diet is a diet that helps prevent malnutrition and noncommunicable diseases. The top U.S. diets include the vegan, TLC, volumetrics, mind diet, DASH, flexitarian, Pritikin, paleo, and the Mediterranean Diet. It is crucial to also include the top U.S. health diets in the mobile health software application because patients also like to include individualized diets that may be a personal choice, not a health bound choice to better their health. For example, Each person's dietary habit is likely to be influenced by various matters, including availability and affordability of food such as meat, fish, vegetables and fruits, lifestyle and work conditions, family habit, social pressure from friends and colleagues, cultural beliefs and traditional customs, personal preference, and lack of nutritional knowledge (Sabila, 2020). The mobile health software application should be fully customizable to allow the combination of both health bound diets, diets caused by a health need or issue, and diet of personal choice to provide the patient with an app that can be fully tailored to their needs to help them create recipes that are custom to what their needs are.

Also, nutrition therapy involves multiple face-to-face sessions over an extended length of time with trained personnel. However, many health care providers cite a lack of education, educational materials, and time to counsel their patients on nutrition. Advancements in technology may be able to circumvent these issues and expand access to nutrition therapies for patients (Kavanagh et al., 2022). It is important for the mobile health software application to provide patients with an efficient way to help give patients the resources they need, such as recipes, to successfully self-manage their diets from home. The mobile health software application can be a solution to this shortage and will make it more accessible for patients to have access to nutritional resources.

The mobile health software application can serve as a more cost-effective method than traditional nutritional therapy. Patients can have more consistent nutritional therapy sessions with better attendance using new emerging technologies to ensure patients have access to dietary resources (Kavanagh et al., 2022). The literature demonstrates the prevalence of noncommunicable diseases and provides statistics of the significance of these diseases (Figure 9). Since noncommunicable diseases are very prevalent in the U.S., it is important to equip patients with educational resources to equip patients to become more independent with their self-management of their dietary health conditions and diets.

Figure 9

United States Nutrition Related Health Conditions

HEALTH CONDITIONS	STATISTICS
Overweight and Obesity	- About 74% of adults are overweight or have obesity. - Adults ages 40 to 59 have the highest rate of obesity (43%) of any age group with adults 60 years and older having a 41% rate of obesity. - About 40% of children and adolescents are overweight or have obesity; the rate of obesity increases throughout childhood and teen years.
Cardiovascular Disease (CVD) and Risk Factors: - Coronary artery disease - Hypertension - High LDL and total blood cholesterol - Stroke	- Heart disease is the leading cause of death. - About 18.2 million adults have coronary artery disease, the most common type of heart disease. - Stroke is the fifth leading cause of death. - Hypertension, high LDL cholesterol, and high total cholesterol are major risk factors in heart disease and stroke. - Rates of hypertension and high total cholesterol are higher in adults with obesity than those who are at a healthy weight. - About 45% of adults have hypertension.[a] - More Black adults (54%) than White adults (46%) have hypertension. - More adults ages 60 and older (75%) than adults ages 40 to 59 (55%) have hypertension. - Nearly 4% of adolescents have hypertension.[b] - More than 11% of adults have high total cholesterol, ≥240 mg/dL. - More women (12%) than men (10%) have high total cholesterol, ≥240 mg/dL. - 7% of children and adolescents have high total cholesterol, ≥200 mg/dL.
Diabetes	- Almost 11% of Americans have type 1 or type 2 diabetes. - Almost 35% of American adults have prediabetes, and people 65 years and older have the highest rate (48%) compared to other age groups. - Almost 90% of adults with diabetes also are overweight or have obesity. - About 210,000 children and adolescents have diabetes, including 187,000 with type 1 diabetes. - About 6-9% of pregnant women develop gestational diabetes.
Cancer[c] - Breast Cancer - Colorectal Cancer	- Colorectal cancer in men and breast cancer in women are among the most common types of cancer. - About 250,520 women will be diagnosed with breast cancer this year. - Close to 5% of men and women will be diagnosed with colorectal cancer at some point during their lifetime. - More than 1.3 million people are living with colorectal cancer. - The incidence and mortality rates are highest among those ages 65 and older for every cancer type.
Bone Health and Muscle Strength	- More women (17%) than men (5%) have osteoporosis. - 20% of older adults have reduced muscle strength. - Adults over 80 years, non-Hispanic Asians, and women are at the highest risk for reduced bone mass and muscle strength.

Note. Facts about nutrition related health conditions in the United States by the U.S. Department of Agriculture & U.S. Department of Health and Human Services. (2020). *Dietary guidelines for Americans, 2020 – 2025.* (https://www.dietaryguidelines.gov/sites/default/files/2021-03/Dietary_Guidelines_for_Americans-2020-2025.pdf). In the public domain.

Health Issues Caused by Poor Diets

Health issues that can be caused by poor diets or lifestyle choices include obesity, cardiovascular disease, diabetes, cancer, bone health, and muscle strength. These types of health issues are noncommunicable diseases, which are health conditions caused by poor habits and can lead to a lifelong health condition (Harvard T.H. Chan School of Public Health, 2023). Noncommunicable diseases are preventable and deciding to make diet changes can reduce a person's risk of getting a chronic disease. Making changes in diet and lifestyle patterns can make a person healthier and prevent chronic disease.

Explanation and Examples of Good Diets

The following paragraphs are explanations and examples of healthy diets that are the top U.S. health diets. The top U.S. diets include the vegan, TLC, volumetrics, mind diet, DASH, flexitarian, Pritikin, paleo, and the Mediterranean Diet. Each diet can provide various health benefits according to the type of health condition. The following explanations also include a suggested diet guide for each of these types of diets. These diet guides can then be used as a foundational resource during the app development.

Vegan. The purpose of the vegan diet is to lose weight and lower cholesterol levels, which can lower the risk of heart disease. The vegan diet is a plant-based diet that focuses on fiber and nutrient dense foods that lowers cholesterol to improve heart health, lower blood sugar levels, reduces cancer risk, and help maintain healthy weight levels (Barnard et al., 2020). This diet should be included in the mobile health software application because it helps lower the risk of the top five noncommunicable diseases. Vegan diets are quite common throughout the U.S. and including this diet will be beneficial since so many people use this as a preventive diet to improve their health. The vegan diet guide is a diet guide to use as a future source to guide the development of the app in the future. Please view the following guide. It is important to know what each diet includes, so when the app is created, the app can accurately create recipes for the different health diets.

Vegan Diet Guide

- Produce: The bright colors you see in the produce aisle reflect different phytochemicals that benefit health, so be sure to choose a variety of fruits and vegetables. Look for fresh herbs, too, which can add flavors and spices to recipes without extra calories and fat.

- Dried Foods: Dried beans and peas, brown rice, whole-wheat pasta, quinoa, barley, oats, cereals, and other whole grains are all great choices.

- Canned Foods: Beans, plant-based soups, and vegetables can all be found in the canned foods aisle. Remember to keep your diet low in sodium and read ingredient lists carefully for animal additives like chicken broth or milk.

- Refrigerated Foods: Tofu, tempeh, hummus, bean- and lentil-based salads, and plenty of non-dairy plant milks and yogurts can be found in this section.

- Frozen Foods: Frozen fruits and vegetables are a wonderful way to save time and money! They are just as nutritious as fresh vegetables and last for much longer. Most stores are also now well stocked with low-fat, frozen plant-based meals like pizzas, pasta dishes, burritos, and veggie burgers. Remember to check labels for hidden animal ingredients, like cheese or egg.

- Follow the Power Plate, an approach that focuses on fruits, vegetables, grains, and beans and sets aside animal products (meat, dairy, and eggs) and added oils.

Note. Vegan Diet Guide, adapted from Physicians Committee for Responsible Medicine. (2020). *Vegan Diet Guide.* (https://pcrm.widencollective.com/portals/gr0kpkol/factsheets).

Paleo. The paleo diet was formed around the idea that people should eat foods that were eaten by early humankind of early hunting and gathering because the human body was not meant to follow the modern diets formed by farming and this can lead to obesity, diabetes, and heart disease. This diet focuses on fruits, vegetables, fish, eggs, nuts, seeds, and lean meats and excludes whole grains, dairy, and refined sugar. Many people who follow the diet hope to optimize their health, decrease risk of chronic disease, and lose weight (Physicians Committee for Responsible Medicine, 2023). The paleo diet should be included in the mobile health software application because it is a preventive diet that leads to better health outcomes and can reduce the risk of obesity, heart disease and diabetes. With diabetes, obesity, and heart disease being such prevalent health issues that many in the U.S. face, this diet should be included in the app. The *Paleo Diet Guide* originates from the Mayo Clinic staff on the Paleo diet; and this guide will be a good resource to use as the basis of the app.

Paleo Diet Guide

What to eat

- Fruits

- Vegetables

- Nuts and seeds

- Eggs

- Lean meats, especially grass-fed animals, or wild game

- Fish, especially those rich in omega-3 fatty acids, such as salmon, mackerel, and albacore tuna.

- Oils from fruits and nuts, such as olive oil or walnut oil.

What to avoid

- Grains, such as wheat, oats, and barley.

- Legumes, such as beans, lentils, peanuts.

- Dairy products, such as milk and cheese.

- Refined and added sugar.

- Added salt.

- Starchy vegetables, such as corn, jicama, peas, and white potatoes.

- Highly processed foods, such as chips or cookies.

A typical day's menu

- Breakfast. Broiled salmon and cantaloupe.

- Lunch. Salad made with romaine, carrot, cucumber, tomatoes, avocado, walnuts, and lemon juice dressing.

- Dinner. Lean beef sirloin tip roast; steamed broccoli; salad made with mixed greens, tomatoes, avocado, onions, almonds, and lemon juice dressing; and strawberries for dessert.

- Snacks. An orange, carrot sticks or celery sticks.

A paleo diet might help manage:

- Weight loss

- Blood pressure

- Cholesterol

- Triglycerides (Mayo Clinic Staff, 2023).

Note. Paleo Diet Guide, adapted from Mayo Clinic Staff. (2023). *Paleo diet: What is it and why is it so popular?* (https://www.mayoclinic.org/healthy-lifestyle/nutrition-and-healthy-eating/in-depth/paleo-diet/art-20111182).

Mediterranean Diet. The Mediterranean Diet focuses on plant-based foods and healthy fats (Figure 10). It has been found to produce healthy heart benefits. According to a study published in 2018, it was found that those who followed the Mediterranean diet over a five-year time span that group had a 30% lower relative risk of cardiovascular events than the low-fat diet group. These events included heart attacks, stroke, or cardiovascular-related death. These benefits are responsible from the healthy fats found in the Mediterranean Diet that come from the consumption of olive oil, nuts, and fish (Cleveland Clinic, 2022). It is beneficial for this diet to be included into the mobile health software application because this diet is important for heart health and produces heart healthy benefits that can improve health outcomes. This diet is an effective way to prevent heart conditions and since heart disease is one of the leading noncommunicable diseases, this diet should be included into the app. The *Mediterranean Diet Guide* can be used in the app as a resource.

Mediterranean Diet Guide

In general, if you follow a Mediterranean Diet, you will eat:

- Lots of vegetables, fruit, beans, lentils, and nuts.

- Lots of whole grains, like whole-wheat bread and brown rice.

- Plenty of extra virgin olive oil (EVOO) as a source of healthy fat.

- A moderate amount of fish, especially fish rich in omega 3 fatty acids.

- A moderate amount of cheese and yogurt.

- Little or no meat, choosing poultry instead of red meat.

- Little or no sweets, sugary drinks, or butter.

- A moderate amount of wine with meals (but if you do not already drink, do not start).

The Mediterranean Diet has many benefits, including:

- Lowering your risk of cardiovascular disease.

- Supporting a body weight that is healthy for you.

- Supporting healthy blood sugar, blood pressure, and cholesterol.

- Lowering your risk of metabolic syndrome.

- Supporting a healthy balance of gut microbiota (bacteria and other microorganisms) in your digestive system.

- Lowering your risk for certain types of cancer.

- Slowing the decline of brain function as you age.

- Helping you live longer.

Food	Serving Goal	Serving Size	Tips
Fresh fruits and vegetables	Fruit: 3 servings per day Veggies: At least 3 servings per day	Fruit: ½ cup to 1 cup Veggies: ½ cup cooked or 1 cup raw	Have at least 1 serving of veggies at each meal. Choose fruit as a snack.

Food	Serving Goal	Serving Size	Tips
			Choose oats, barley, quinoa, or brown rice.
Whole grains and starchy vegetables (potatoes, peas, and corn)	3 to 6 servings per day	½ cup cooked grains, pasta, or cereal; 1 slice of bread; 1 cup dry cereal	Bake or roast red skin potatoes or sweet potatoes. Choose whole grain bread, cereal, couscous, and pasta. Limit or avoid refined carbohydrates.
Extra virgin olive oil (EVOO)	1 to 4 servings per day	1 tablespoon	Use instead of vegetable oil and animal fats (butter, sour cream, mayo). Drizzle on salads, cooked veggies, or pasta. Use as dip for bread. Add salads, soups, and pasta dishes.
Legumes (beans and lentils)	3 servings per week	½ cup	Try hummus or bean dip with raw veggies. opt for a veggie or bean burger.
Fish	3 servings per week	3 to 4 ounces	Choose fish rich in omega-3s, like salmon, sardines, herring, tuna, and mackerel. Ideally, choose walnuts, almonds, and hazelnuts.
Nuts	At least 3 servings per week	¼ cup nuts or 2 tablespoons nut butter	Add cereal, salad, and yogurt. Choose raw, unsalted, and dry roasted varieties. Eat alone or with dried fruit as a snack.

Food	Serving Goal	Serving Size	Tips
Poultry	No more than once daily (fewer may be better)	3 ounces	Choose white meat instead of dark meat. Eat in place of red meat. Choose skinless poultry or remove the skin before cooking. Bake, broil or grill it.
Dairy	No more than once daily (fewer may be better)	1 cup milk or yogurt; 1 ½ ounces natural cheese	Choose naturally low-fat cheese. Choose fat-free or 1% milk, yogurt and cottage cheese. Avoid whole-fat milk, cream, and cream-based sauces and dressings. Limit egg yolks.
Eggs	Up to 1 yolk per day	1 egg (yolk + white)	No limit on egg whites. If you have high cholesterol, have no more than 4 yolks per week.
Red meat (beef, pork, veal, and lamb)	None, or no more than 1 serving per week	3 ounces	Limit to lean cuts, such as tenderloin, sirloin, and flank steak.
Wine (optional)	1 serving per day (people assigned female at birth) 2 servings per day (people assigned male at birth)	1 glass (3 ½ ounces)	If you don't drink, the American Heart Association cautions you not to start drinking. Talk to your healthcare provider about the benefits and risks of consuming alcohol in moderation.
Baked goods and desserts	Avoid commercially prepared baked goods and desserts.	Varies by type	Instead, choose fruit and nonfat yogurt. Bake using liquid oil instead of solid fats; whole grain flour instead of bleached or

Food	Serving Goal	Serving Size	Tips
	Limit homemade goods to no more than 3 servings per week		enriched flour; egg whites instead of whole eggs.

Note. Mediterranean Diet Guide, adapted from Cleavland Clinic. (2022). *Mediterranean diet.* (https://my.clevelandclinic.org/health/articles/16037-mediterranean-diet).

Figure 10

Mediterranean Diet Checklist

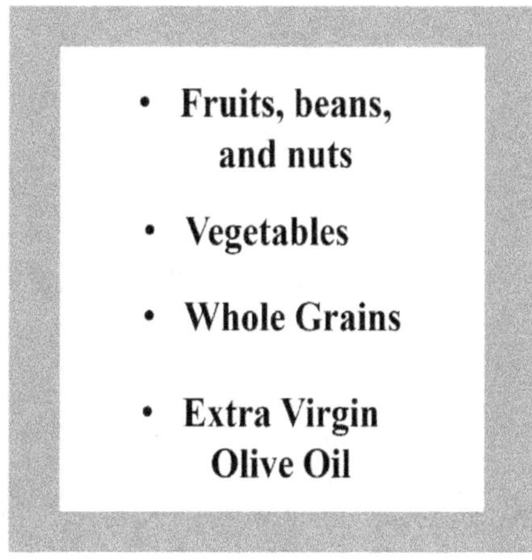

Note. Plan your meals around these foods for a Mediterranean Diet, adapted from Cleveland Clinic. (2022). *Mediterranean diet checklist.* (https://my.clevelandclinic.org/health/articles/16037-mediterranean-diet).

Pritikin.   The Pritikin diet's purpose is to minimize the amount of processed foods consumed. This diet focuses on high fiber and unprocessed foods. It can help improve heart disease and lose weight. In particular, the Pritikin Diet discourages animal and plant fats high in saturated fats, which are linked to poorer heart health in some studies. Still, the diet encourages foods high in omega-3s, which are a type of unsaturated fat linked to improved heart and brain health (Division of Global Health Protection, Global Health, Centers for Disease Control and Prevention, 2023). This diet will be included in the mobile health software application because it is a holistic and preventive method to improve heart health and lose weight. Also, 67 participants attended the Pritikin Longevity Center for 12–15 days and experienced an average 3% decrease in their body mass index (BMI), as well as a 10–15% decrease in blood pressure and cholesterol levels (Division of Global Health Protection, Global Health, Centers for Disease Control and Prevention, 2023). This diet should also be included into the app because there is research from the literature that shows it is an effective diet that can improve health outcomes. The *Pritikin Diet Guide* is a diet guide that is attached to use as a future resource for the app.

Pritikin Diet Guide

Food lists:

The Pritikin Diet has a clear and organized list of foods to eat, limit, or avoid. Foods to eat are labeled *go* foods, while foods that should be limited or avoided are *caution* and *stop* foods. You are also encouraged to get most of your protein from plant-based foods, such as tofu, edamame, beans, peas, and lentils. Furthermore, if you are trying to lose weight, you are advised to eat unlimited vegetables and high fiber foods (e.g., cooked oatmeal, brown rice) and limit higher calorie foods, such as nuts, seeds, breads, and crackers.

Foods on the *go* list include:

- Fruits and vegetables (4–5 servings of each per day): aim for a variety of colors and types; eat them in their whole form either fresh, frozen, or canned without syrup

- Complex carbs (5 or more servings per day): whole grains (whole wheat breads and pastas, brown rice, oatmeal, rye, quinoa, barley, millet, etc.), starchy vegetables (potatoes, sweet potato, yams, winter squashes, etc.), and legumes (black beans, kidney beans, chickpeas, lentils, peas, etc.)

- Nuts and seeds: limit servings to no more than 1 ounce (28 grams) per day

- Dairy (2 servings per day): nonfat cow's milk, nonfat yogurt, and fortified soymilk

- Lean protein (no more than one serving per day): skinless white chicken or turkey, lean red meat (bison, venison), and a large emphasis on plant-based proteins, such as legumes and soy products (tofu, edamame)

- Fish (no more than one serving per day): fresh or canned (unsalted) fatty fish, such as salmon, sardines, herring, mackerel, and trout

- Eggs: up to two servings of egg whites per day (no yolks); you may have more than two servings if this replaces other animal proteins

- Beverages: water as your main beverage; no more than 400 mg of caffeine per day from unsweetened tea (preferably green or herbal tea) or filtered coffee (removes diterpenes that may increase LDL (bad) cholesterol)

- Artificial sweeteners: no more than 10–12 packets of Splenda or Stevia each day

- Herbs, spices: all herbs and spices are allowed and should replace added sugar, fat, and salt

Foods to avoid:

Foods that should be avoided completely or limited to once per month include:

- Animal fats and processed oils: butter, chicken fat, chocolate, coconut oil, cocoa butter, hydrogenated and partially hydrogenated vegetable oils, lard, margarine, palm oil, palm kernel oil, shortenings, etc.

- Processed and high fat meats: organ meats and processed meats (e.g., bacon, sausage, ham, bologna)

- Whole fat dairy: all cheeses, cream cheese and other processed varieties, whole fat milk, whole fat yogurt, sour cream, etc.

- Nuts: only coconuts should be avoided due to their high saturated fat content

- Other foods: egg yolks, fried food or foods cooked in oil, nondairy whipped toppings, high fat pastries and desserts, salty snack foods, etc.

The Pritikin Diet emphasizes whole, unprocessed foods that are low in fat and high in fiber. Approximately 10–15% of calories should come from fat, 15–20% from protein, and 65–75% from complex carbs. The plan is based on a stoplight system with a list of *go, caution,* and *stop* foods. *Go* foods include fruits, vegetables, whole grains, starchy vegetables, legumes, fish, lean protein, and low fat, calcium-rich foods like fat-free yogurt. *Caution* foods should be limited, but you can still eat them on occasion. These include oils, refined sugars (e.g., syrups and fruit juices), and refined grains (e.g., white bread, pasta, and rice). Finally, *stop* foods should be eaten no more than once per month and include animal fats (e.g., butter), tropical oils (e.g., coconut oil), processed oils (e.g., hydrogenated margarine), organ and processed meats, whole fat dairy, and processed treats.

Note. Pritikin diet review: Benefits, downsides, and more, adapted from Davidson, K. (2020). *Pritikin diet review: Benefits, downsides, and more.* (https://www.healthline.com/nutrition/pritikin-diet-review).

DASH.   The DASH diet was created to lower blood pressure and LDL *bad* cholesterol and to produce more heart healthy outcomes. This diet controls hypertension and provides goals, rather than requiring special foods. This diet prevents heart conditions from occurring by encouraging healthy eating habits that can reduce blood pressure levels (National Heart, Lung, and Blood Institute, 2021). This diet should be included in the mobile health software application because it prevents high blood pressure from occurring and this can lead to patients having more healthy hearts and reduce their risk of heart disease. The *DASH diet guide* will serve as a valuable resource for the mobile health software application to know the guidelines of the diet (Figure 11).

DASH Diet Guide

This plan recommends:

- Eating vegetables, fruits, and whole grains.

- Including fat-free or low-fat dairy products, fish, poultry, beans, nuts, and vegetable oils.

- Limiting foods that are high in saturated fat, such as fatty meats, full-fat dairy products, and tropical oils such as coconut, palm kernel, and palm oils.

- Limiting sugar-sweetened beverages and sweets.

When following the DASH eating plan, it is important to choose foods that are:

- Low in saturated and trans fats.

- Rich in potassium, calcium, magnesium, fiber, and protein.

- Lower in sodium

Note. DASH Diet Guide, adapted from **National Heart, Lung, and Blood Institute. (2021).** *DASH eating plan.* (https://www.nhlbi.nih.gov/education/dash-eating-plan).

Figure 11

DASH Eating Plan

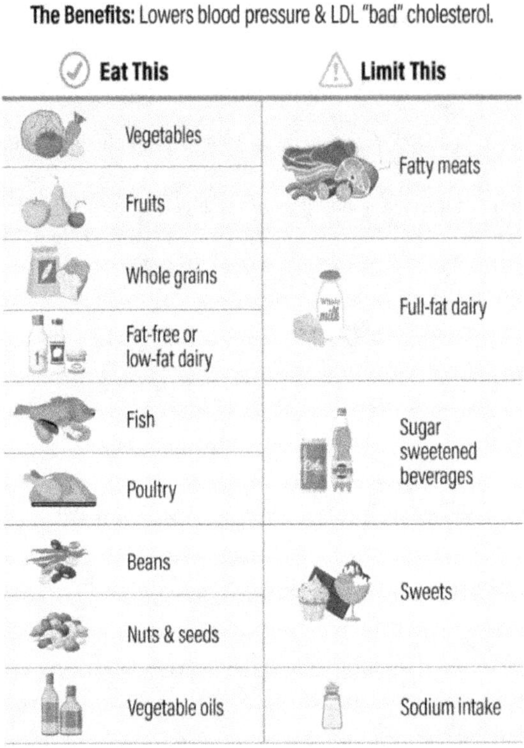

The Benefits: Lowers blood pressure & LDL "bad" cholesterol.

✓ Eat This	⚠ Limit This
Vegetables	Fatty meats
Fruits	
Whole grains	Full-fat dairy
Fat-free or low-fat dairy	
Fish	Sugar sweetened beverages
Poultry	
Beans	Sweets
Nuts & seeds	
Vegetable oils	Sodium intake

Note. A guide of which foods to consume and limit, by the National Heart, Lung, and Blood Institute. (2021). *DASH eating plan.* (https://www.nhlbi.nih.gov/education/dash-eating-plan). In the public domain.

Flexitarian. The purpose of the flexitarian diet is to eat natural foods. This diet focuses on increasing the daily consumption of fruits and vegetables; and focuses on eating natural foods that are not processed or genetically modified. This diet does not focus on calorie counting and it focuses on eating the most natural ingredients. The benefits of this diet are to lose weight, decrease the risk of heart disease, diabetes, and cancer (Patton, 2021). This diet will be included in the mobile health software application because it leads to beneficial health outcomes, and it is a holistic way for patients to reduce their risk of noncommunicable diseases. The flexitarian diet is one of the top U.S. diets and since it is so popular with patients, it should be included (Patton, 2021). The *Flexitarian Diet Guideline* can be used as a guiding resource for the app. This can be a useful resource because it will help with the app development, to know which foods can be eaten for which diet.

Flexitarian Diet Guideline

The flexitarian diet is made to be inclusive, but you do want to limit animal protein (including seafood) and processed foods and beverages. Here is what to add to your shopping cart.

Load up on:

- Fruits and vegetables.

- Plant proteins (beans such as black, kidney or navy, edamame, chickpeas, lentils, tofu).

- Whole grains (brown rice, oats, barley, quinoa).

- Plant-based milk (although dairy milk is OK in moderation).

- Eggs and dairy (cheese, yogurt, or dairy alternatives).

- Nuts, nut butters, seeds, and healthy fats. Oils, herbs, and spices.

Limit:

- Meat and poultry (lean cuts of beef, chicken breast, turkey breast).

- Fish (salmon, tilapia, cod, shrimp).

- Anything with added sugar or refined carbohydrates

Note. Flexitarian Diet Guide, adapted from **Cleveland Clinic**. (2021). *What is the flexitarian diet?* (https://health.clevelandclinic.org/what-is-the-flexitarian-diet/).

TLC. The purpose of the TLC diet is to lower cholesterol levels. This diet adopts a heart healthy eating plan to better improve heart health of patients. This diet is a simpler version of the DASH diet, and it ensures you eat each nutrient from the categories. The aim of the TLC diet is to help you eat healthier foods, cooked in healthier ways. This is not a temporary diet, but rather a new way of eating that is both heart healthy and tasty. What you eat greatly affects your blood cholesterol levels and adopting a heart healthy eating plan—one that is low in saturated fat, trans fat, and cholesterol is key to this diet (National Heart, Lung, and Blood Institute, 2005). Since the TLC diet is a simpler version of the DASH diet, this diet should also be included in the mobile health software application as a heart disease diet (Figures 12.1 and 12.2).

Figures 12.1 and 12.2

TLC Diet Guideline

BOX 19

Eating Well With TLC

The TLC Diet calls for a variety of foods that are low in saturated fat, trans fat, and cholesterol but high in taste. It is not a deprivation diet. It can satisfy your taste buds as much as your heart. Here's the breakdown of the TLC diet by food groups (see Box 33 on page 55 for a guide to serving sizes):

Breads/Cereals/Grains	**6 or more servings a day—adjust to calorie needs** *Foods in this group are high in complex carbohydrates (see Box 20 on page 36) and fiber. They are usually low in saturated fat, cholesterol, and total fat.* Whole-grain breads and cereals, pasta, rice, potatoes, low-fat crackers, and low-fat cookies
Vegetables/Dry Beans/Peas	**3–5 servings a day** *These are important sources of vitamins, fiber, and other nutrients. Dry beans/peas are fiber-rich and good sources of plant protein.* Fresh, frozen, or canned—without added fat, sauce, or salt
Fruits	**2–4 servings a day** *These are important sources of vitamins, fiber, and other nutrients.* Fresh, frozen, canned, dried—without added sugar
Dairy Products	**2–3 servings a day—fat free or low fat (for example, 1% milk)** *These foods provide as much or more calcium and protein than whole milk dairy products—but with little or no saturated fat.* Fat-free or low-fat milk, buttermilk, yogurt, sour cream, cream cheese, low-fat cheese (with no more than 3 grams of fat per ounce, such as low-fat cottage cheese)
Eggs	**2 or fewer yolks per week—including yolks in baked goods and in cooked or processed foods.** Yolks are high in dietary cholesterol. Egg whites or egg substitutes have no cholesterol and less calories than whole eggs.

Meat/Poultry/Fish	**5 or less ounces a day**
	Poultry without skin and fish are lower in saturated fat. Lean cuts of meat have less fat and are rich sources of protein and iron. Be sure to trim any fat from meat and remove skin from poultry before cooking.
	Lean cuts of beef include sirloin tip, round steak, and rump roast; extra lean hamburger; cold cuts made with lean meat or soy protein; lean cuts of pork are center cut ham, loin chops, and pork tenderloin
	Strictly limit organ meats, such as brain, liver, and kidneys—they are high in cholesterol.
	Eat shrimp only occasionally—it is moderately high in cholesterol.
Fats/Oils	**Amount depends on daily calorie level**
	Nuts are high in calories and fat, but have mostly unsaturated fat. Nuts can be eaten in moderation on the TLC diet—be sure the amount you eat fits your calorie intake.
	Unsaturated vegetable oils that are high in unsaturated fat (such as canola, corn, olive, safflower, and soybean); soft or liquid margarines (the first ingredient on the food label should be unsaturated liquid vegetable oil, rather than hydrogenated or partially hydrogenated oil) and vegetable oil spreads; salad dressings; seeds; nuts.
	Choose products that are labeled "low-saturated fat," which equals 1 gram of saturated fat per serving.
Diet Options:	
Stanol/sterol-containing food products (see pages 27–28)	Specially labeled margarines and orange juice
Soluble fiber	Barley, oats, psyllium, apples, bananas, berries, citrus fruits, nectarines, peaches, pears, plums, prunes, broccoli, brussels sprouts, carrots, dry beans, peas, soy products (such as tofu, miso)

Note. A TLC diet chart by the National Heart, Lung, and Blood Institute. (2005). *TLC diet guideline.* (https://www.nhlbi.nih.gov/resources/your-guide-lowering-cholesterol-therapeutic-lifestyle-changes-tlc). In the public domain.

Mind Diet.   The purpose of the MIND diet is to focus on brain healthy foods that can reduce the risk of developing dementia. Although the main purpose is to promote brain health, it is also beneficial to reduce cardiovascular disease. This diet is effective because the Rush Memory and Aging Project (MAP) collected data for 10 years on older participants that followed this diet, and it was found to be effective. Also, more than 1,000 participants filled out annual dietary questionnaires for ten years and had two cognitive assessments. A MIND diet score was developed to identify foods and nutrients, along with daily serving sizes, related to protection against dementia and cognitive decline. The study showed that participants that were following the MIND diet had a slower rate of cognitive decline than participants that did not follow the diet. The effects of the MIND diet on cognition showed greater effects than either the Mediterranean or the DASH diet alone (Harvard T.H. Chan School of Public Health, 2023). This diet should be included in the mobile health software application because it is an effective way to prevent brain diseases and can lead to better cognitive health outcomes. The *MIND Diet Guideline* is a diet guideline that can be used as a future resource for the app.

MIND Diet Guideline

- 3+ servings a day of whole grains

- 1+ servings a day of vegetables (other than green leafy)

- 6+ servings a week of green leafy vegetables

- 5+ servings a week of nuts

- 4+ meals a week of beans

- 2+ servings a week of berries

- 2+ meals a week of poultry

- 1+ meals a week of fish

- Mainly olive oil if added fat is used

The unhealthy items, which are higher in saturated and trans-fat, include:

- Less than 5 servings a week of pastries and sweets

- Less than 4 servings a week of red meat (including beef, pork, lamb, and products made from these meats)

- Less than one serving a week of cheese and fried foods

- Less than 1 tablespoon a day of butter/stick margarine (Harvard T.H. Chan School of Public Health, 2023).

Note. MIND Diet Guide, adapted from **Harvard T.H. Chan School of Public Health.** (2023). *Diet review: MIND diet.* (https://www.hsph.harvard.edu/nutritionsource/healthy-weight/diet-reviews/mind-diet/).

Volumetrics. The purpose of the volumetrics diet is to promote wight loss by providing recommendations to eat filling, low calorie foods that are dense in nutrients. This diet recommends eating lots of healthy foods that are low in calories, and it can help people eat healthier foods, while still being able to lose weight (Cleveland Clinic, 2022). This diet can be included into the mobile health software application because it can be used as a preventive way to prevent obesity and lose weight. Since obesity is another main noncommunicable disease, this diet will be important to include. The *Volumetrics Diet Guideline* is a diet guideline that will be good to use as a future resource in the creation of the app.

Volumetrics Diet Guideline

The Volumetrics diet breaks food down into four categories. To determine which category a food

belongs in, you divide the number of calories per serving by its weight in grams. The result is a

number between zero and nine. If you are attempting to lose weight on the Volumetrics diet, you

are encouraged to eat 1,400 calories a day. The majority of what you eat in a day should come

from categories one and two, but occasional, small indulges from categories three and four are

acceptable (Cleveland Clinic, 2022).

1.   Category one (calorie density under 0.6): This category of food forms the foundation of

your diet. In other words, this is the stuff you fill up on. These foods — due to their high-water

content — should help you feel full. A few examples of category one foods are:

- Fruits like bananas, apples, and grapefruit.

- Non-starchy vegetables like broccoli, carrots, beets, and Brussels sprouts.

- Nonfat dairy products like nonfat yogurt or skim milk. (If you are not a dairy drinker, never

  fear: Most unsweetened milk substitutes also fall into this category.)

- Broth-based soups of all sorts.

2.   Category two (calorie density 0.7 to 1.5): This category contains foods that are healthy

when consumed in moderation. A few examples of category two foods are:

- Skinless chicken and turkey and lean cuts of pork or beef.

- Legumes: lentils, chickpeas, and dried beans.

- Starchy vegetables: corn, potatoes, and squash.

- Whole grains: brown rice, quinoa and farro.

3.   Category three (calorie density 1.6 to 3.9): This category contains food that, while still fairly healthy, should only be consumed in small portions. A few examples of category three foods are:

- Fatty meat and fish, as well as skin-on poultry.

- Full-fat dairy products such as ice cream, cheese, and whole milk.

- Refined carbohydrates like pasta, white bread, and white rice.

4.   Category four (calorie density 4 to 9): This category includes processed, sugary, and fatty foods, which should be eaten very sparingly. A few examples of category four foods are:

- Nuts and seeds.

- Oils, butter and shortening.

- Fast food, candy, and chips.

In addition to the dietary measures, the Volumetrics diet recommends getting 30 to 60 minutes of exercise per day.

Note. Volumetrics Diet Guide, adapted from Cleveland Clinic. (2022). *What is the volumetrics diet?* (https://health.clevelandclinic.org/volumetrics-diet/).

Sample Example Recipes

The mobile health software application will create custom recipes based upon the patient's health conditions and will combine all diet restrictions to generate individualized recipes. The patient will also have an option to choose serving size, food likes and dislikes, along with cultural food preferences. Also, it was found the results of this pilot study demonstrated increased motivation in participants to make dietary changes and improve personal health, drawing attention to the importance of considering culturally tailored health interventions (Sijangga et al., 2023). The mobile health software application will include cultural preferences into the app. Food is a main component of culture and incorporating it into the app will increase app utility and engagement since it can be personalized to the patient's needs. The patient can choose whether they would like it to generate an appetizer or snack, main meal recipes, dessert, or drinks, or be a holiday themed dish. As part of the mobile health software application research, sample example recipes and sample menus by health condition will be found in appendix D. Please refer to appendix D to view the sample menus and recipes.

Mental Health Diets

Including mental health diets into the mobile health software application will be a good diet to include because mental health is increasing in need; and mental health and diet are closely related. For example, there is a growing body of evidence indicating that nutrition may play a key role in the prevention, development, and management of diagnosed mental health problems including depression, anxiety, schizophrenia, Attention Deficit Hyperactivity Disorder (ADHD) and dementia. Clinical studies point to the importance of diet as one part of the jigsaw in the prevention of poor mental health and mental health problems and the promotion of positive mental health and brain development (Mental Health Foundation, 2017). The literature uncovered there is a need to include mental health diets into the app and many sources found that as more people are diagnosed with mental health conditions, they need help from a nutritionist to help formulate diet plans for them.

Also, unhealthful dietary patterns that typically lead to obesity, diabetes, and other physical health problems can contribute to poor mental health. Several studies show that people who follow a Western diet comprising highly processed foods are more likely to have major depression or persistent mild depression. People who follow a Mediterranean diet, on the other hand, seem to be less likely to have mental health conditions (Caporuscio, 2019). Including mental health diets can better assist patients because diet can reduce the symptoms of mental health conditions and can

serve as a holistic and lower cost method to manage mental health symptoms. If a person is missing

certain nutrients it can lead to a deficiency that can cause mental health symptoms and it shows

which foods are good food sources for these nutrients (Figure 13). Please see Appendix E to view

the mental health diet guide.

Figure 13

Essential Vitamins and Minerals.

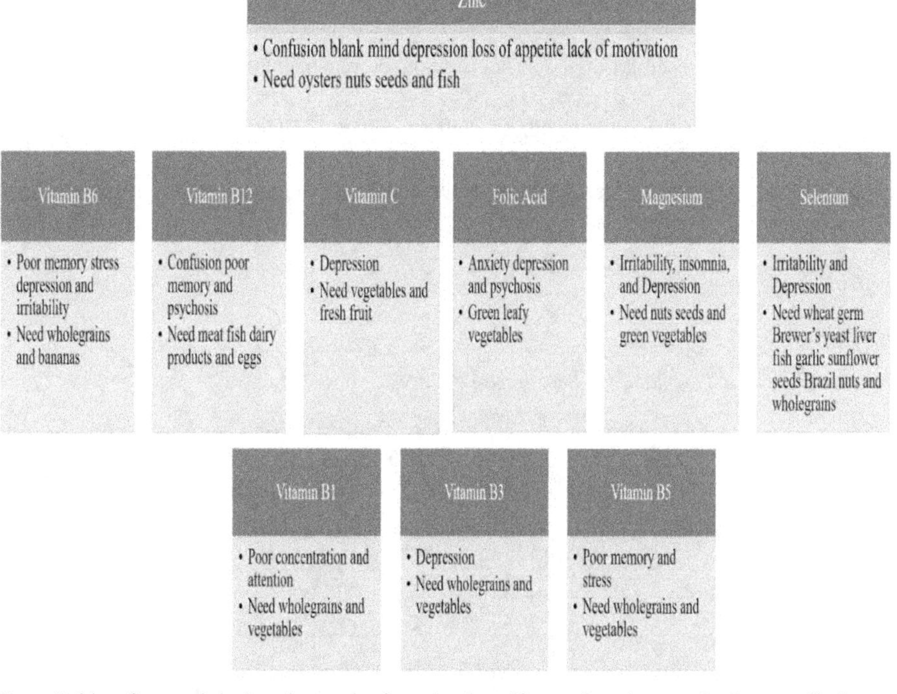

Note. Table of essential vitamins and minerals, the effects of various and where to find them. Adapted from Mental Health Foundation. (2017). (https://www.mentalhealth.org.uk/sites/default/files/2022-04/food-for-thought-mental-health-nutrition-briefing-march-2017.pdf).

Literature that Supports the Problem: A Lack of Healthcare Resources and a Nutritionist Shortage

It is imperative for businesses to invest in the innovation of digital healthcare solutions to assist patients in navigating their health management for long term chronic conditions. Chronic diseases result in 7 out of 10 deaths among Americans each year and account for 75 percent of the nation's health spending, according to the Centers for Disease Control and Prevention. Proper nutrition, health screenings and other preventive measures cannot only reduce these deaths but save billions in health care costs each year. There will be a national shortage of RDNs by 2020 and the field will experience 16 percent growth in job opportunities between 2014 and 2024 (Cooper, 2019). There is a great need for digital health technology implementation in the healthcare sector to help assist and bridge the gap in healthcare staffing (Figure 14). Digital health technologies can be a useful tool for healthcare staff to use to increase adherence rates of patient self-management care.

Figure 14

Projected Supply and Demand for Registered Dietitians

	Scenario One (Status quo)	Scenario Two (Evolving care delivery)
Supply		
Estimated supply, 2016	78,970	78,970
Projected supply, 2030	97,940	97,940
New entrants, 2016-2030	58,200	58,200
Attrition[a], 2016-2030	-39,230	-39,230
Projected supply, 2030	97,940	97,940
Total growth (%), 2016-2030	18,970 (24%)	18,970 (24%)
Demand		
Estimated demand, 2016	78,970	78,970
Projected demand[e], 2030	95,540	99,540
Changing demographics, 2016-2030	16,570	16,570
Achieving population health goals	NA	4,690
Increased managed care	NA	1,010
Avoidable hospitalization and ED use	NA	-1,700
Total growth (%), 2016-2030	16,570 (21%)	20,570 (26%)
Projected Supply (minus) Demand, 2030	**2,400**	**-1,600**

Notes: All numbers reflect full time equivalents (FTEs). Numbers may not sum to totals due to rounding. NA denotes "not applicable".

Note. Projected Supply and Demand for Registered Dietitians in the United States, 2016 – 2030, by the HRSA Health Workforce. (2016). Registered Dietician Data. (https://bhw.hrsa.gov/sites/default/files/bureau-health-workforce/data-research/registered-dieticians-2016-2030.pdf). In the public domain.

Healthcare staff may not be always there with the patient, but incorporating digital health technologies into the continuity of care can assist in better patient communication and data accuracy to see how patients are doing, and to prevent a health issue from occurring. With rising health care costs, an aging population, and anticipated physician shortage, there is a pressing need for innovative advances in health technology. Funding agencies are increasingly interested in supporting research that can quickly benefit patients (Siefert et al., 2019). The mobile health software application will help fill the shortage by producing an innovative solution for patients to receive custom tailored recipes according to their long-term conditions, allergies, or noncommunicable diseases. The mobile health software application will alleviate the burden of the nutritionist shortage by creating an app that can help patients create recipes and will help them with diet adherence using preventive care techniques. Patients will no longer need to wait for long wait times to see a nutritionist to create custom food recipes for their daily needs.

As the population ages, there will be a greater population of society that will have multiple noncommunicable diseases. Demographic trends indicate that the proportion of the world population over the age of 60 will double from 11% now to 22% by 2050 (El – Kour et al., 2021). When patients are diagnosed with new health conditions, they are not educated on how to eat for the long term. This requires hospitals to sponsor patient educational programs, which can be very costly, time consuming, inequitable to rural communities, and only a few patients can attend due to maximum capacity. As the need for nutritionists or dietitians increases, there is a decrease of students receiving terminal degrees in this field, resulting in a larger shortage (Figure 15). It is estimated there will be a national shortage of 1,600 RDNs by 2030 (Joo et al., 2022). The mobile health software application will be a much more inexpensive method to provide support to patients at home and help them adhere to their diets by providing them with custom generated recipes. The mobile health software application can be a more accessible and low-cost method for public health and healthcare organizations to use as a preventive care tool. This is useful to use because it will make it easier for patients to eat healthily and will lead to a reduction in health complications.

Figure 15

Academy of Nutrition and Dietics Data Show that Only 3% of RDNs Hold a Terminal Degree

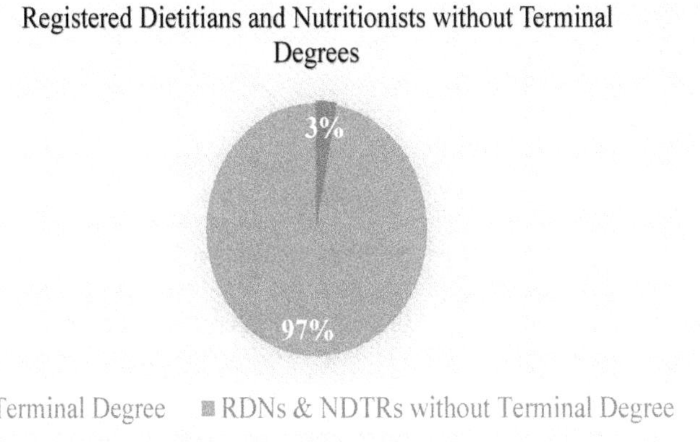

Note. The shortage of registered dietitians or nutritionists with a terminal degree: A call to action for the profession. Adapted from Academy of Nutrition and Dietetics. (2023). (https://doi.org/10.1016/j.jand.2023.01.003).

Literature that Supports the Solution

Educating and Supporting the Healthcare Consumer Using Mobile Apps

Mobile apps can be a significant technological advancement in the healthcare industry. Utilizing apps as a method in patient interventions can lead to great benefits. Mobile health (mHealth) is a rapidly growing research field that aims to study the effect of mobile phone-based interventions on health and behaviors. The advantages of mHealth solutions include less personnel resources and the possibility to access intervention content at any time and wherever the user is.

In addition, mHealth interventions provide great flexibility in terms of translation and modifications to provide inclusive content and features (Alexandrou et al., 2021). Developing the mobile health software application will assist patients in their self-management of noncommunicable and chronic diseases. Before creating a business proposal, it is important to first examine best practices and gaps in the literature that will provide supporting evidence for the mobile health software application.

Examining the literature, it was found that apps can improve public health and support self-management by providing patients with mobile health interventions without having to wait for their next appointment. There is a greatly significant p – value between knowledge, general, and specific diet (Figure 16). This shows there is a need for an intervention that will assist patients in better understanding and managing their noncommunicable and chronic illnesses for improved self-management of care.

Figure 16

Paired Sample T Test on Self – Efficacy, Knowledge, and Self – Management, Exploring Changes in Self-Efficacy, Knowledge and Self-Management in Only the High and Mid Users of Capability

Outcome	Pretest, mean (SD)	Posttest, mean (SD)	Change Score	T - Test	P - Value	Cohen d
Self – Efficacy	3.25 (0.9)	3.86 (0.75)	0.61	-3.13	0.008	0.74
Knowledge	0.82 (0.14)	0.85 (0.11)	0.03	-1.25	0.23	0.24
General Diet	3.82 (2.38)	4.96 (1.37)	1.14	-2.46	0.29	0.59
Specific Diet	3.14 (1.51)	3.82 (1.20)	0.68	-1.66	0.12	0.50
Exercise	1.54 (2.14)	2.75 (1.86)	1.21	-2.93	0.01	0.60

Blood Glucose	3.61 (3.25)	4.61 (2.83)	1.00	-1.88	0.08	0.33
Foot Care	4.22 (2.70)	4.54 (2.08)	0.32	-0.67	0.51	0.13

Note. Incorporating behavioral trigger messages into a mobile health app for chronic disease management: Randomized clinical feasibility trial in diabetes. Adapted from JMIR mHealth and uHealth. (2020). (https://doi.org/10.2196/15927).

When a patient gets diagnosed for the first time with a health condition, they are not aware and have enough knowledge about their condition to properly utilize self-management techniques. Also, mHealth apps can provide users with extensive educational material to improve self-efficacy and to simplify behavior change. The creation of population-based spark triggers for chronic disease could be an effective approach to cueing positive behavioral tasks for large populations at a time through mHealth. This could become a powerful tool that could be utilized in accountable care organizations, managed care organizations, large health care systems, or population health management at any level (JMIR mHealth and uHealth, 2020). Healthcare professionals have limited time to educate the patient about it, and they send them home with a printout fact sheet, nutritional guide, or set them up with educational classes that can conflict with the patient's working hours.

Apps can help reduce the barriers of conflicting schedules, limited time, a shortage of healthcare professionals, and access to transportation by providing an alternative method to education that can be accessed anywhere at any time without needing to schedule a prior appointment. By 2025, nearly three-fourths of all internet users will access the web exclusively by mobile phone. This increasing reliance on mobile phones has sparked the creation of self-help health apps, known as mobile health (mHealth). They aim to improve public health by supporting patient-led self-care (Krzyzanowski et al., 2020). Using mobile apps can improve accessibility to healthcare resources, especially for rural areas or for patients who lack access to transportation.

The advantages of using apps along with primary care is it can increase accessibility and it can increase communication, so healthcare providers can check in with their patients before waiting to see their patients at their next yearly checkup. To further develop an understanding of mobile apps, the topics of how to create an app creation guide, examples of different health app case studies, and evaluating the app effectiveness with health outcomes will further be discussed.

Effectiveness of Mobile Apps

How to Create an App - A Mobile Health App Creation Guide. This part of the research will examine and provide a basic overview of the steps that will be needed to create the mobile health software application. Mobile app development is rapidly growing. For organizations to be successful, they must meet user expectations by developing mobile applications that fit their customers' expectations (IBM, 2023). Developing a customized recipe app generator can help patients better adhere to their chronic condition's diets. It is important before building the business proposal to examine the literature on how the mobile health software application can be created. It is important to do this to first consider the feasibility of the app, before building the business proposal.

When developing an app, you need to know how to break the app idea into various categories or domains to help you create the best app possible. You need to recognize the different domains that must all come together to make an app. In this first step, begin thinking about the app in terms of each of the following domains: app idea, key ingredients, concept deign and user experience, technology and development, compliance, and privacy by design, and testing and quality improvement (Salter, 2022). The following steps will help give an overview of the process of what the mobile health software application will entail and what it is visualized as. Following the app creation steps that were found in the literature and then applying it to the mobile health software application will show how the above steps can be applied to this research project.

Steps. The following are an outline of steps guided by Salter's (2022) outline, *From Ideation to Implementation: Steps to a Successful App.*

1. **App Idea.** This step involves determining if you have the needed skills, tools, and equipment to develop an app.

   The beginning idea is: A custom recipe generator app that will generate recipes based on your custom diet constraints based on your health conditions such as food allergies, chronic diseases, noncommunicable diseases, and mental health diets.

   My skills are: Nontechnical skills such as digital and graphic design, branding, marketing, concept design, and end user trials such as budgeting, project management, marketing, overall design, and making business decisions.

   I cannot do: Technical skills such as coding and programming of languages, architecture, development environments, native and hybrid platforms web technologies, network infrastructure, and hardware technology.

   I need to find: A business partner or app developer that understands the technical components.

   Needed tools and equipment: computers, development environment, programming language, version control system, frameworks, Adobe™, and Google Analytics™.

2. **Key Ingredients.** This step involves listing app features, identifying the target user, and creating the 4 w's. App features will help determine what makes your app stand out from the rest of the competition, identifying who your target user will be is important to know who your audience is so you know who you will be solving the problem for, and creating the 4 w's will help you understand your user and their needs.

App Features:

Necessary Features:

- Creates custom recipes based on personalized diet constraints.

- Have a family section to input multiple users to combine everyone's diet constraints to cook one family meal.

- Include a likes/ dislikes section along with cultural food preferences.

- Save your favorite recipes.

- Choose serving size options.

- Includes seasonal and holiday recipes.

- Includes main meals, snacks, desserts, appetizers, and drink recipes.

Nice to have Features:

- Input your nutritional intake to ensure you are meeting recommended U.S. dietary guidelines.

- Basic cooking videos teach you how to cook.

- Available in multiple languages.

- What is in your pantry? – Input ingredients you already have at your home to create recipes with.

- Area to add the ingredients you need for generated recipes in a shopping list.

- Push notification shopping reminders.

The Four W's – Are the target market and help understand who your end user is. Consists of who, why, where, and when. Which domain/target market? For what is the app going to be used? How does the domain affect the app? What are user expectations and is there a niche market to fill? Is there a need for this app? (Salter, 2022).

- **Who (target user):** People of all ages who have multiple chronic, noncommunicable diseases, diet constraints, or food allergies.

- **Why:** Patients need an easier method of creating recipes that align with their health condition's diets.

- **Where**: At home use or healthcare organizations.

- **When:** Before cooking meals.

- **Notes:** Accessibility, inclusive design, and patient centric focus are a priority to eliminate nutritional resource barriers to patients.

3. **User Centered Concept Design and User Experience**. Stakeholders are a vital part of the app deveolpment process because a developer first needs to focus on how the app will affect stakeholders, and anticipate their needs to design the app around their needs. Stakeholders can include patients, healthcare providers, healthcare research instutions, the public, governement agencies, and policy

makers. The mobile health software application will impact healthcare providers and staff by potentially increasing diet adherence rates and leading to better health outcomes. The app can affect public health and governemental agencies by resulting in less heatlhcare spending because patients will not suffer from health complications by adhering to their diets and healthier communities. It will affect patients by leading to better health outcomes and saving time by generating receipes faster than the patient can research it. It can affect healthcare research insitutions because as there is an increased shortage in healthcare professionals, healthcare organizations will further rely on mobile health interventions that can be deveoped by research institutions (Figure 17).

Figure 17

Evidence from the evolution of mobile apps during COVID-19

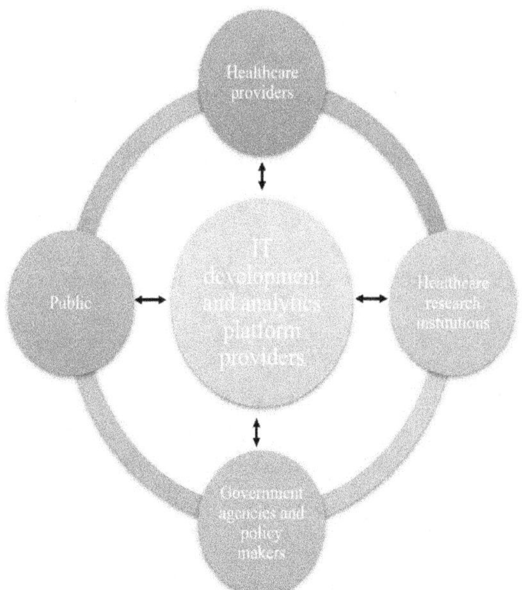

Note. Evidence from the evolution of mobile apps during COVID-19. Adapted from Science Direct. (2021). (https://doi.org/10.1016/j.jbusres.2021.06.002).

Value proposition and problem modeling is important in app development because the more valuable an app is, the better engagement rates it will have, since it solves a problem for the user (Figure 18). People will adopt an innovative technology or product if they can clearly see how, it will improve their lives, without extra effort on their part. Making end users the focal point, starting from design concept to implementation, will increase usability and engagement to improve health outcomes of the users. Human-centered design fits technology into people's existing habits and behaviors and develops solutions to people's problems. Focusing on key values and personalization can achieve a human centered design by thinking how tools provide access, save time, simplify, reduce anxiety, offer motivation and value (Elevance, Health 2022). For an app to be successful, it must provide users with value and be easy for the user to interface with. Applying value proposition to the mobile health software application will provide value to the patients by addressing the problem of time and knowledge constraints in diet adherence to chronic conditions. The mobile health software application makes it easier for the patient to adhere to their diets by generating custom recipes for them to use based on their health conditions. It will help patients save time because patients will no longer spend countless hours researching and creating their own recipes that align with their health conditions. Using new emerging technologies can reduce errors of dietary self-management. If a patient lacks health literacy about their condition and tries to create their own recipes by themselves with an inaccurate understanding of their condition, then this can lead to diet errors that can negatively impact their health.

Figure 18

A proposed framework for product-service system business model design

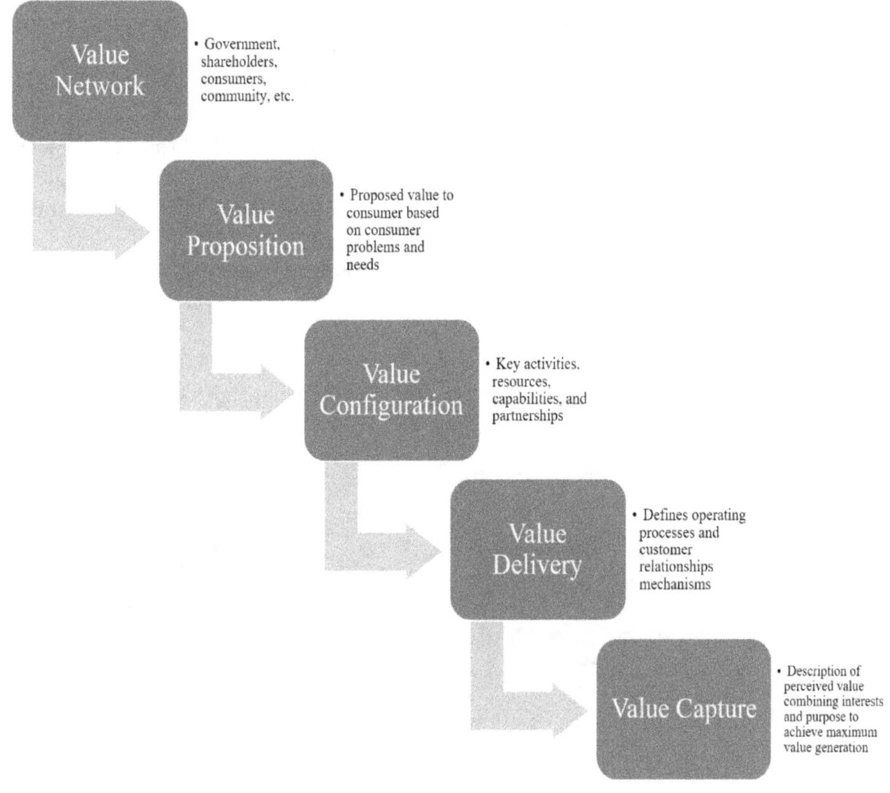

Note. A proposed framework for product-service system business model design. Adapted from Science Direct. (2022). (https://doi.org/10.1016/j.jclepro.2022.134365).

User engagement can determine the success of an app. Apps that typically have higher engagement rates are more likely to be successful. User engagement rates can be driven by a valuable experience that can result in behavioral responses from the user. Effeort, performance, and brand trust are all significant drivers of functional value in an app (Figure 19). Social value can be impacted by networking, enjoyment, and social image. Both functional and social value variables can result in statistically significant user enganegement with mobile health apps that can result in a long term behavior change that leads to user loyalty and advocacy. It is important to consider these variables during the deveopment process of the mobile health software application to plan for long term retention rates of the user. The Appendix G1 table shows that mobile health apps can improve the quailty of life and produce better heatlh outcomes and it is statisically significant. This is vital to discover this in the literature because it shows that this will be a successful and useful intervention that can help patients before building the business proposal.

Figure 19

Building User Engagement to mhealth Apps From a Learning Perspective: Relationships Among Functional, Emotional, and Social Drivers of User Value

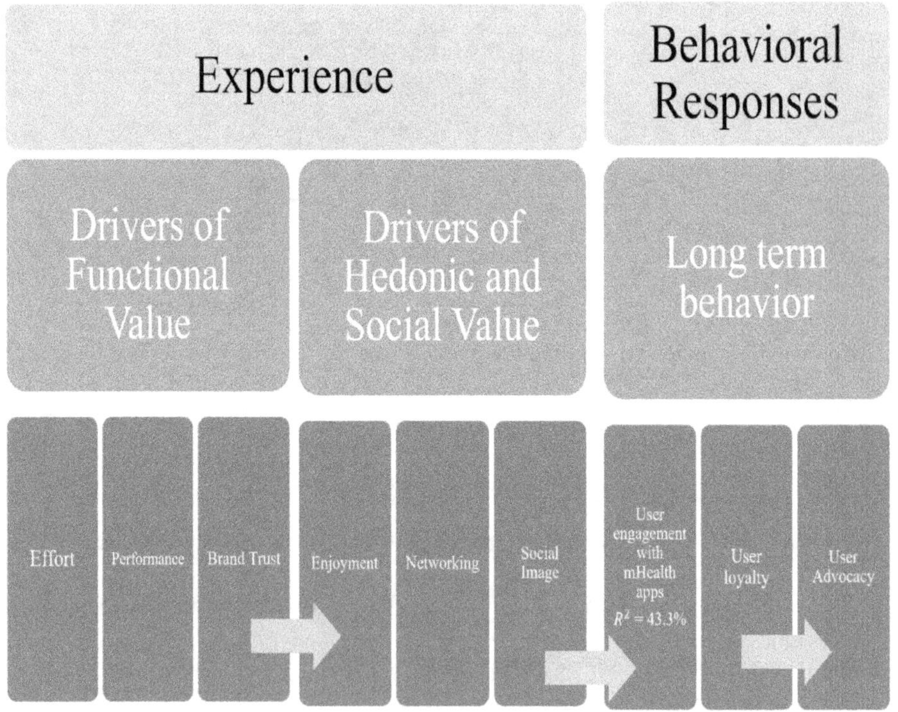

Note. Building user engagement to mhealth apps from a learning perspective: Relationships among functional, emotional, and social drivers of user value. Adapted from Science Direct. (2022). (https://doi.org/10.1016/j.jretconser.2022.102956).

4. **Technology and Development.** This step includes selecting which type of platform and programming language to use. There are three types to choose from native apps, hybrid apps, or web apps. The programming and markup languages used for this kind of software development include Java™, Swift™, C#™ and HTML5™ (IBM, 2023). The mobile health software application will be a native app, since it has the highest satisfaction weighted health app score located in Appendix G2. Native apps are also accessible and have easy user navigation but can have a more expensive startup cost.

5. **Compliance, Privacy by Design, and HIPPA Considerations.** All health care organizations or mobile health apps will be impacted by HIPPA. It is crucial that the mobile health software application is HIPPA compliant since it deals with patient sensitive information. HIPAA IT compliance addresses how data is implemented, maintained, and monitored to safeguard electronic protected health information (ePHI). This specifically addresses the HIPAA Security Rule and should implement authentication measures with security risk assessment to safely store data (Kiteworks, 2022). Since the mobile health software application will be dealing with sensitive patient information, it needs to incorporate privacy by design and implement methods to protect patient information during the app design process. Privacy needs to be a top priority and considering it from the beginning of the design will allow for maximum security, rather than considering security as an afterthought.

Examining the literature, it was found that privacy by design is the most effective way to implement security into health apps. It was found that privacy by design is growing in popularity because patients want to see increased methods of protection and designing an app around privacy most appeals to users. For example, privacy-preserving software solutions help meet regulatory requirements and increase user acceptance by working with and storing anonymized, when possible, minimally necessary sensitive data while respecting user's privacy. Only relevant information should be stored. It is invasive to collect and store unnecessary data against it violates ethical standards used in clinical practices. Therefore, mHealth apps should only store necessary data (Perez et al., 2023). An integral part of the healthcare industry is to do no harm, better known as non-maleficence and creating safety measures can protect the patients and serves as an example of maleficence, doing right to the patient by actively protecting them. It is important for the mobile health software application to protect its users because it is the right thing to do, and it is the industry standard to take an ethical approach.

Using privacy by design method will also increase user trust of the app brand since they can see that the app was designed with protection of privacy as one of the main priorities. Privacy by design can be created by allowing users to choose which data they allow for the app to store. The data collection and storage processes can be decoupled, which allows for the collected data to be processed kept as long as it is necessary before it is discarded (e.g., location data used to determine presence at a certain place). Sensitive data should use a foreground service that will notify the user that the app is using the AwarNS Framework, only while data is being collected in the background (Perez et al., 2023). The literature suggests incorporating these health information security methods and these are transparent methods that can achieve user protection that will achieve HIPPA compliance. These security methods will be incorporated into the mobile health software application to achieve HIPPA compliance and ensure that the users will be provided with protection of their information. The following checklist is a HIPPA IT compliance checklist that the mobile health software application can use as a guiding resource for privacy and compliance.

HIPAA IT Compliance Checklist:

- Have a dedicated HIPAA Privacy Officer responsible for developing and implementing security measures.
- Identify which data is under HIPPA.
- Educate all staff on HIPAA laws and regulations.
- Create and document administrative, technical, and physical policies.
- Ensure all equipment has necessary safety measures.
- Securely store health related documents to limit access to only those the patient agrees to have access to.
- Use encryption software to protect data.
- Practice secure web browsing and use email security software.
- Properly disposing of documents and records containing patient data, shredding, or burning are the preferred, most secure methods.
- Create security breaches procedures.
- Review access logs for unauthorized access.
- Implement comprehensive user logging and auditing procedures.

- Create and use backup procedures that comply with HIPAA guidelines.

- Develop and maintain a contingency plan and disaster recovery system.

Note. Everything you need to know about HIPAA compliance. Adapted from Kiteworks. (2022). (https://www.kiteworks.com/hipaa-compliance/hipaa-compliance-requirements/).

6. **Testing and Quality Improvement.** This step is an iterative process and testing, and quality improvement processes can lead to a better developed app that is of higher quality. This is important to include because having a better developed app will result in higher user satisfaction rates and can lead to an increased trust level between the users and the app. Efficiency, flexibility, reuse, quality, and reliability of the app are all interconnected variables that affect each other and are a significant theme that was identified in the literature to focus on when doing app testing and quality improvement (Figure 20). This applies to the mobile health software application because it is important to offer a high-quality app that patients can efficiently use and customizable to the patients' needs to improve user satisfaction with the app (Salter, 2022, pp. 3 – 4).

Figure 20

Venn Diagram Represnts the Overlapping Studies in Common Goals Attainments

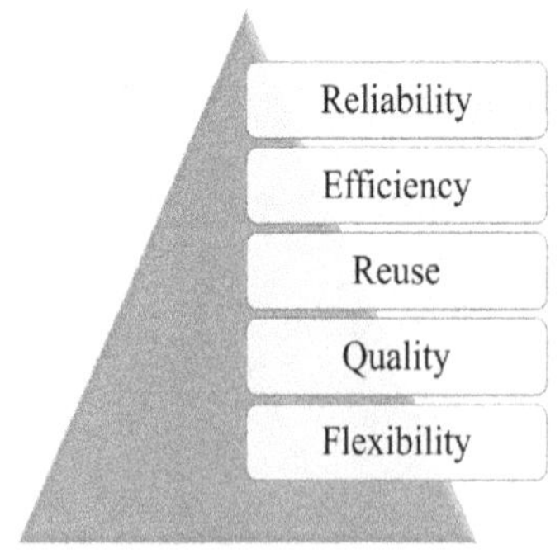

Note. Developing mobile applications via model driven development: A systematic literature review. Adapted from Science Direct. (2021). (https://doi.org/10.1016/j.infsof.2021.106693).

Overview of Successful Apps (Case Studies)

Examining the literature of different types of healthcare apps will give a beneficial analysis of features that will be beneficial to incorporate or lessons to learn from each case study. In a case study for an app that measures the nutritional intake of a user, a focus group was conducted to receive feedback from users. Several features of mobile apps, such as feedback mechanisms, goal setting, peer motivation, and health-related news updates can motivate users to perform new healthful behaviors. Also, mobiles can be a timely device for users to reach the activation threshold as a result of automated prompt message (Ahn et al., 2019). It will be beneficial to incorporate app notifications in the mobile health software application to increase user engagement rates. Also, when patients are busy, notifications can remind patients of their self-management of their diets and can help them achieve their nutritional goals. Challenges of dietary assessment methods are memory reliance, time limitation, skilled staff, knowledge of diets and foods, and other time-consuming tasks. Although complete automation of diet analysis has not been achieved yet, mobile technologies have the potential to improve real-time assessment of the diets of individuals and groups by incorporating their daily dietary routines (Ahn et al., 2019). The mobile health software application will reduce these burdens by making it accessible for anyone from any educational background to better adhere to their noncommunicable or chronic conditions diets. Instead of taking an intensive amount of time to research all your diets and try to find recipes that can adhere to them by researching for countless hours, the mobile health software application will take all diets into consideration and generate recipes that will align with your conditions.

In another case study, for a pediatric healthcare app, a focus group was conducted to receive feedback from patients and healthcare providers. It was found that parents need resources to assist them in their self-management of care for their child that has chronic conditions. Parents shared their challenges they faced when supporting their child's health behaviors, they emphasized a need for a personalized app, and want more accessible ways to access app content (audio/video). Nurses emphasized the need of supporting parents early, and the value of a shared platform in different languages, to facilitate communication. This study highlights the needs of parents and how adding audio, and video files can fulfill parental and increase accessibility (Alexandrou et al., 2021). According to this focus group feedback, it will be beneficial if the mobile health software application includes these components to the design of the app to better assist the patients. The focus group feedback uncovers that there is a gap in care and parents need more resources to better manage their kids' chronic conditions.

The mobile health software application can be tailored to the patients by making it customizable to their health conditions and generating recipes according to their diets. The app can create custom generated recipes on a digital recipe card, but according to this focus group feedback the app should also include videos to demonstrate cooking techniques to help first time parents navigate through learning how to cook for their kids. Also, to increase patient accessibility to nutritional resources, the app should be available in the U.S. top languages such as English, Spanish, and Chinese; until there are more resources or an identified need to expand the app to more languages. Latino people are the fastest and largest growing minority group in the U.S. and are projected to account for one-third of the US population by 2060 with high rates of chronic conditions. The Centers for Disease Control and Prevention reported that 14.2% of Latinos had two or more concurrent chronic conditions. Health information technology (IT) tools are increasingly being used within health care settings and have been proven to enhance patient-provider communication and lead to better health outcomes. However, English-only health IT tools could potentially increase health disparities if they only benefit English speakers. Therefore, developing culturally responsive Spanish-language health IT tools is imperative (Ruvalcaba et al., 2019). A lot of app developers focus on creating English only apps but making it more accessible through languages can expand the number of users and can gain a competitive edge in the marketplace. Also, local nutritionists or dietitians in the patient's area may not understand their language and creating a nutritional app that can be accessible to all types of languages can help local healthcare providers in serving them.

Patients have limited access to nutritional resources and lack education about their chronic conditions. Healthcare organizations and public health must look to mobile health app technologies to provide patients with nutritional support to have patients better adhere to their diets, and result in better health outcomes. Many patients became frustrated with accessing information and struggled to find reliable diet information. Although there are dietitians available, patients wish to have continuous access to information about food selection. Patients reported using the internet as the most accessible and most convenient platform for answers regarding diet, despite knowing that it could lack accuracy (El Khoury et al, 2019). This case study example describes there is a need for nutritional intervention to further support patients of their self-management of chronic diets and patients struggle to educate themselves on their diets. Having an assigned nutritionist or dietitian is not enough support for patients because they are not available most of the time, and the shortage of healthcare professionals that are trained in nutrition is limited since there is a shortage of registered dietitians. This case study describes that patients are open to using the internet as a resource since nutritional printouts are not informational, easily accessible, and are time consuming with limited food choices. This case study example can be applied to the mobile health software application because it supports that patients will be supportive of using a digital resource and there is a need for this app. The mobile health software application will be a valuable resource for healthcare organizations to adopt because it will increase patient satisfaction, accessibility of resources, and can provide better diet adherence which can lead to better patient rates for the health organizations.

A case study on a mobile health app intervention for cardiovascular health in African Americans discovered that health disparities can be reduced in the African American community and mobile health app interventions can provide effective and more accessible resources. For example, prior studies have pointed to multiple barriers such as fatigue, time, cost, and lack of social support leading to poor diet and PA among African Americans. Overall, there was an improvement in perceived barriers to healthy diet, which further correlated with improvements in dietary intake. These findings suggest that our mHealth lifestyle intervention may offer support to African Americans in the navigation of perceived barriers stemming from longstanding structural inequities by providing education and highlighting practical strategies to incorporate healthy diet into daily life (Cyriac et al., 2021). The mobile health software application can assist in resolving these barriers by using digital app technologies to provide more accessible and equitable nutritional self-management resources. It is vital that all patients receive the opportunity to properly self-manage their chronic conditions. Educating patients about their conditions is critical in self-management because if a patient is not informed enough of how to care for their condition, this can result in irreversible health complications, a lower quality of life, and reduced years of life. Adhering to diets is a form of preventative care and can result in better health outcomes. The mobile health software application can reduce this barrier because patients will no longer have to struggle to educate themselves on how to adhere to their diets and it will create custom recipes that patients can follow.

App Effectiveness with Health Outcomes

Mobile Health (mhealth) intervention apps are found to be effective in providing improved health outcomes in patients. It was found in an intervention study in Japan to reduce obesity that mobile apps do result in improved health outcomes and weight loss. Mobile health (mHealth) interventions, a more cost-effective approach compared with traditional methods of delivering lifestyle coaching in person, have been shown to improve physical parameters and lifestyle behavior among overweight populations (Kondo et al., 2022). This Japanese intervention study supports that apps can effectively improve health outcomes in patients.

Also, it was found in a meta-analysis of 47 randomized controlled trials that health apps support patients and lead to improved health outcomes. Web-based interventions in primary care settings improved risk factors for cardiovascular disease compared with standard of care alone. Thus, health apps can provide an alternative and complementary approach to delivery of preventive nutrition therapy within the limits of primary care, where the shift to remote care during the COVID-19 pandemic has further highlighted the need for evidence-based health apps (Kavanagh et al., 2022). Now more than ever before, health apps can help address the shortage of healthcare professionals and can lead to a solution for an increasing population that has chronic conditions, and a shorter supply of nutritionists and dietitians.

Health apps can also increase accessibility in rural areas. It was found in a Hawaiian nutritional case study, that an increased utilization of resources like nutritional support may improve the primary care shortages seen in Hawaii, particularly in rural areas and for populations that are disproportionately affected by health disparities (Joo et al., 2022). Using the mobile health software application in rural areas can help address patients who cannot access nutritional support, because they lack dietitians or nutritionists in their areas.

These three studies show that apps can effectively produce better health outcomes in patients, and it is a significant solution that will provide patients with a valuable resource; and result in directly correlated improved health outcomes for their self-management of chronic or noncommunicable diseases. As health care costs rise, insurers will look to dietitians for affordable and targeted preventive care (Cooper, 2019). The mobile health software application can provide health organizations with a less expensive form of preventive care and help improve diet adherence rates in their patients. Now that we have examined that health apps do result in improved patient outcomes, the literature shows that the mobile health software application can be an effective intervention for patients to better support and provide them with custom recipes that will lead to improved diet adherence and improved health outcomes.

Theoretical Framework: Business Theories and Concepts

Throughout the research, I have identified several business theories that can be beneficial to the research of app development. I considered theories that are focused on business technology startups or theories that are founded in entrepreneurial mindset that I found from the literature. I will further compare these theories to identify the best business model theory to use as the framework and basis of the research. I will compare the strengths and limitations of all concepts or theories to further identify which ones should be incorporated into the research and to be used as the foundational model of this research. Overall, the best theory and concept to use are the business plan theory with a patient centric approach and the strategic management concepts that focus on purpose to frame the development of this app. This theory and concept are chosen because the business plan incorporates all major aspects of business concepts, and it has been used as the golden standard for decades and strategic management was chosen because it is crucial to form strategies of how the business will establish and keep its competitive edge against its competitors in the industry for short- and long-term goals, while considering a purpose driven strategy. Having a solid business plan and creating short- and long-term strategies will give the company direction and is the key to success for any business.

Strategic Planning Model

Strategic management is a concept that was created in the 1960's by Chandler, Ansoff, and Andrews. The purpose of strategic management is to continuously develop goals that the organization wants to achieve, methods of action that will give the best competitive edge in the market and dedicate resources to achieve these goals. The primary function of any organization is value creation, especially in transformative industries such as healthcare (Schiavone et al., 2021). Value creation is a type of strategic management. It is a crucial aspect of an organization because for patients to come back and be loyal to the organization, the organization must deliver and create a service of value that meets the needs of the patients. From the patient's perspective, an organization that gives them greater value and benefit will be the organization that has a competitive advantage in the market because more patients want to go there since it is of greater value than the competitors.

Using multiple strategies in a strategic plan is crucial because there are a lot of moving variables, and each variable may need a different type of strategy to accomplish short- and long-term goals. Different types of strategic management include the implementation strategy, better known as the balanced scorecard, value creation strategy, mass customization, stakeholder analysis, SWOT analysis, and a competitor analysis (Ginter et al., 2018). Every goal is unique, and using different strategies can be used to better fit every type of situation and give a greater competitive advantage. Unanticipated events can occur and using different types of strategies can lead to greater flexibility to handle these changes.

Close cooperation and patient centricity prove useful not only for improvements of services but also to create value within the community. Furthermore, the case study findings demonstrate that the actors in the healthcare ecosystem can produce high-quality service solutions by considering the digitalization of their business models (Schiavone et al., 2021). Focusing on digitalization of healthcare resources in the mobile health software application will better assist the patient in self-management of noncommunicable diseases by providing them with resources and support to adhere to their noncommunicable diets to improve their health outcomes. Digitalizing the way patients can create dietary recipes custom to their conditions is a type of strategic value because patients no longer must wait, and they can access new recipes at any location or time and save time researching new recipes. Digital health should be ethical, secure, and accessible. It should be developed with principles of transparency, accessibility, scalability, replicability, interoperability, privacy, security, and confidentiality (World Health Organization, 2021). The mobile health software application will also address privacy issues as a strategy to establish trust with patients and healthcare providers.

Some strategic concepts that the mobile health software application will incorporate into the business plan includes the implementation strategy, better known as the balanced scorecard, value creation strategy, mass customization, stakeholder analysis, SWOT analysis, and a competitor analysis. These strategies have been chosen to be utilized in the research because it focuses on all aspects of the business, and it will create and identify short and long-term goal strategies to further differentiate the app against the competitors.

General Business Theories

The Golden Circle. The golden theory was created by Simon Sinek in 2009, when he presented it during one of his TED[TM] talks (Figure 21). Sinek is a marketing consultant, and he created this theory from his own experiences, and he uses human decision making as one of the main concepts in his theory. The golden circle theory explains that for businesses to be successful or create a valued service or product, they must understand their purpose and be able to explain how their product or service brings value and has a unique market differentiation to make their product or service stand out amongst their competitors.

Figure 21

Golden Circle Theory

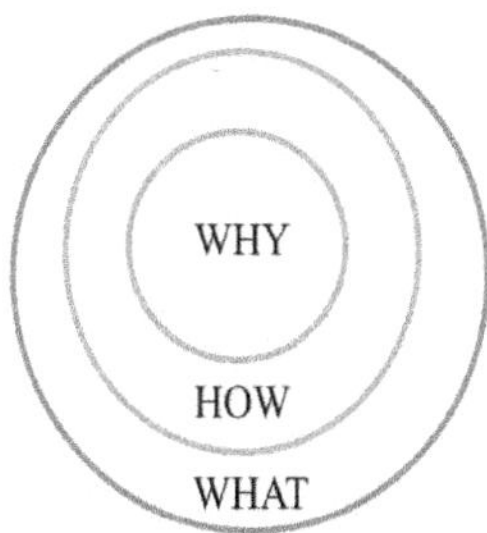

Note. Customized adjuncts with clear aligner therapy: The golden circle model explained! Adapted from Journal of the World Federation of Orthodontists. (2022). (https://doi.org/10.1016/j.ejwf.2022.10.005).

The theory describes that most professionals know *WHAT* they are doing, some know *HOW* they do it, and few professionals know *WHY* they are doing it. *WHY* is the purpose of taking action. Rather than think from the outside in, Sinek states successful leaders use inspiring stories and think from the *inside out* from *WHY* to *WHAT* (Journal of the World Federation of Orthodontists, 2022). The strengths of this theory include that it is purpose driven and has a focus on a larger cause. This is important to have because the healthcare industry has an extremely patient centric focus. Healthcare organizations tend to prioritize and put the patient first to meet the needs of the patient and to improve their level of care. The golden circle keeps brand messaging consistent, provides direction, and differentiates the organization.

The limitation of this theory is the majority of healthcare organizations already use a patient centric focus and this is the new industry standard to have, and it does not differentiate them to stand out as much. It is the new industry standard, and it is a basic expectation for healthcare organizations to care about their patients and to see them as people who need help and not to see them as a means to an end. It is the basic responsibility for all healthcare organizations to uphold the concepts of non-maleficence, do no harm, and beneficence, do good. Also, this model focuses too much on the why, but loses sight and excludes the who of whom the target audience is. To be able to succeed, the healthcare organization must first focus on who their target demographic is and then focus on the patient's needs and problems before attempting to address a purpose. Although it is crucial to incorporate a purpose forward driven approach into an organization, there are other theories or concepts that can be used to accomplish this. This theory will not be used for the mobile health software application due to its limitations and it is a newer theory that needs to be further developed; and a mission statement can provide the same consistent brand messaging and provide direction to the organization. Purpose driven strategic concepts also will be another superior concept to use because it focuses on both short- and long-term goals, where the golden circle model does not consider both.

Ansoff Matrix. Igor Ansoff developed the Ansoff Matrix in 1957 and it analyzes the risks and benefits a certain strategic decision brings (Figure 22). Ansoff is known as the father of strategic management. The Ansoff matrix is a fundamental business framework taught worldwide and it is used to measure the attractiveness of leveraging existing products and markets vs. new ones, as well as the level of risk associated with each. Products are located on the X-axis and markets are located on the Y-axis. Each matrix indicates a specific growth strategy such as market penetration, the concept of increasing sales of existing products into an existing market, market development, focuses on selling existing products into new markets, product development, focuses on introducing new products to an existing market, and diversification, the concept of entering a new market with altogether new products (Peterdy, 2023).

Figure 22

Ansoff Matrix

	Existing Products	New Products
Existing Markets	Protect and Build	Product Development
New Markets	Market Development	Diversification

Note. Ansoff matrix: In the procurement models handbook (3rd ed.). Adapted from Routledge. (2019). (https://doi.org/10.4324/9781351239509-14).

The strengths of the Ansoff matrix include that it is easy to use, it includes short- and long-term planning, analyzes the level of risk, and considers all alternatives. It is important to use a simple tool because it will be easier for all levels of employees to understand and there is less risk of error when using it. It is also important for businesses to consider both short term and long-term goals to provide the organization with direction during decision making. Analyzing the level of risk is important for the organization to know, before deciding to make an investment on a decision. Considering all alternatives is important for organizations to be well informed, weigh all actions, and pick the best decision that will help the company in their mission and vision.

Limitations to this theory include that competitors are ignored, it lacks a cost benefit analysis, and it is difficult to predict consumer and market behaviors. Ignoring competitors is a large limitation because to maintain a competitive edge, all businesses or organizations must keep track of each other and develop new strategies to grow the business and keep their edge over their competitors. If an organization does not do this, then they will lose out on profits and go out of business because they are not maintaining or creating a new product differentiation strategy. Lacking a cost benefit analysis is another significantly large limitation because if you cannot measure the effectiveness of a new strategy being implemented, then you do not know if it is beneficial for the organization to pursue or if it is a waste of resources. Since it is hard to predict the matrix's effectiveness on consumer and market behaviors, then this tool is risky and is not a stable tool to use. When an organization or company is considering using a method of measurement, it is important to choose a tool that is consistent to make the most out of the company's resources.

This tool is not a useful tool to use for the healthcare industry or for the mobile health software application because the majority of healthcare organizations have extremely limited resources, and it is imperative to have a method of key performance indicators that measure how the strategies perform. The healthcare industry is extremely competitive, and this tool will not be an effective tool in the industry because it ignores analyzing the competitors; healthcare organizations are always researching the competitors to find new ways to stand out. This theory will not be used for the mobile health software application and rather a SWOT analysis will serve as a better tool to use because it considers the competitors, it is a reliable and low-cost tool, it is easy to understand and uncovers competitive advantages in a neutral way and provides key market insights on an industry.

Business Model Canvas. The business model canvas was created by Alex Osterwalder, an entrepreneur and business theorist, in 2005. The business model canvas gives a quick overview of nine core business components that feature how the organization will deliver value and operate.

It is a one-page summary of the business plan and serves as a visual graphic and provides easy comprehension of the business. The main nine components are depicted (Figure 23).

Figure 23

Business Model Canvas

Key Partners	Key Activities	Value Proposition	Customer Relationships	Customer Segments
	Key Resources		Channels	
Cost Structure			Revenue	
Social and Environmental Costs			Social and Environmental Benefits	

Note. The case for a socially oriented business model canvas: The social enterprise model canvas. Adapted from Journal of Social Entrepreneurship. (2019). (https://doi.org/10.1080/19420676.2018.1541011).

The strengths of this model include that it is a very visual, easy method of communication, and gives a quick overview of the core business components in a concise and easily understandable manner. The canvas is a tool used by entrepreneurs to communicate their business venture ideas with one another in a time efficient manner (Ripsas et al., 2018). The business model canvas is a helpful tool when pitching a new company idea or giving a basic overview presentation.

The limitations of the business model canvas includes that it does not picture the business environment that influences the organization, it does not give a clear method of how to foster innovation for new startups, and it does not include strategic methods. BMC was characterized as 'static' because it does not capture changes in strategy or the evolution of the model. It limits the focus on the organization, and it isolates the organization from its environment, whether this is related to industry structure or to stakeholders, such as society and natural environment (Sparviero, 2019). Not focusing on external factors such as the environment of the industry and stakeholder's needs is a large limitation because the healthcare industry is very much impacted by the environmental structure and environment of the economy. In this research project, noncommunicable diseases are greatly impacted by external forces and ignoring these external factors will be a detriment not to consider. Noncommunicable diseases are very much impacted by external factors such as patient's behaviors, innovative technology, public health programs, access to care, and new disease outbreaks just to name a few. The business model canvas will not be a good theory to use for the mobile health software application because it does not include the external forces of healthcare, it lacks incorporation of strategy into business operations, and it needs to go more in depth of the startup and be more researched and well thought out. Also, to secure funding a traditional full length business plan will need to be created, and it is more efficient to develop a full-length business plan to conserve resources and to be time efficient.

Business Plan or Business Proposal. The business plan was created by Pierre Samuel, a mill business entrepreneur, in 1799. The purpose of the business plan is to provide investors with a roadmap of your company's goals and how it will achieve them, along with including a summary of the business and its financials and basic business information. The business plan is a valuable tool for raising capital, finding strategic partners, recruiting, and providing an internal guide on how to drive a company's growth (Figure 24). The plan should be concise, well written, and dynamic. The business plan is an operational roadmap that tests an organization's vision and strategy. It also serves as an important communication document when seeking investment in the business (Conrad et al., 2019). The business plan is an industry standard for any organization, and it is used worldwide with an organized and highly detailed document that covers all aspects of a

business.

Figure 24

Key Elements of a Business Plan

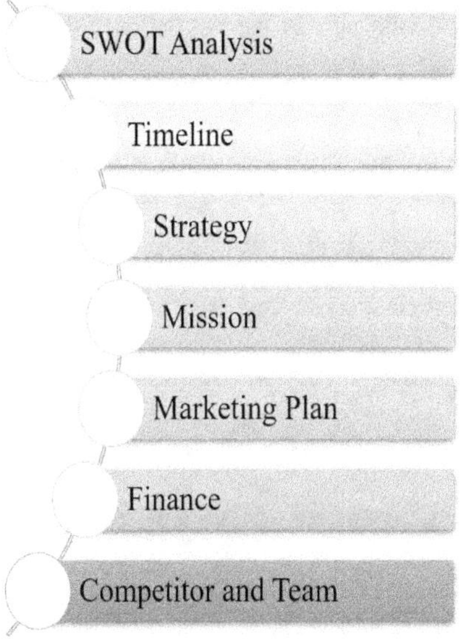

Note. 12 Key elements of a business plan (top components explained). Adapted from
Founder Jar. (2022). (https://www.founderjar.com/elements-of-business-plan/).

The limitation of this theory is that it does not place the patient or consumer at the center

of development. A common business plan pitfall includes focusing only on the product without

framing it in the context of the consumers/patients (Conrad, 2019). It is important to keep a patient

centric focus because the more centered it is around the patient, the more utility and value it will

add. Although this is a limitation, the business plan has the fewest limitations and it will be the

best overall theory to use for the mobile health software application, alongside incorporating

strategic management and a patient centric approach to the business plan.

Strengths of the business plan includes that it uncovers business weaknesses before the

business is launched, it identifies potential opportunities, it analyzes the market and industry, it incorporates strategy, serves as a step-by-step plan, and calculates how much startup capital will

be needed. The business plan is a detailed blueprint that you can refer to during the startup process

and helps you maintain your momentum (Score Foundation, U.S. Small Business Administration,

2023). When creating a business plan for a new organization or already existing one, a business

plan keeps business owners organized on the next steps that need to be achieved and it documents

how you will achieve them. Business owners can become overwhelmed and formulating a

business plan keeps them accountable and on track for their short term and long-term goals and

vision. Developing and using a business plan is statistically significant and is a proven traditional

working method to start a business (Figure 25). These findings suggest that entrepreneurs should

engage in some lean startup activities and still write a business plan (New England Journal of

Entrepreneurship, 2021). Using a business plan to develop the mobile health software application

will be a great foundational theory to use as the basis of my research because it is statistically

significant, and the business plan has been used as the industry standard of many successful

businesses for several decades.

Figure 25

Business Plans and Lean Startup

Business Plans and Lean Startup	
Variables	Summary Regression Results of Success
Business Plan	0.09
Lean Startup	0.09

Note. The road to entrepreneurial success: Business plans, lean startup, or both? Adapted from New England Journal of Entrepreneurship. (2021). (https://doi.org/10.1108/NEJE-08-2020-0031).

Chapter 3 - Methods

The purpose of this study is to develop a business proposal for a mobile healthcare application using a business plan format and strategic management concepts as the theoretical framework. The research will uncover potential competitors in the market and will review user feedback to discover attributes that can lead to a competitive advantage in the market. This chapter will cover the research design, research setting, methods, sample frame, sample size, and data collection methods. This chapter will also explain data analysis methods, the Institutional Review Board process, (IRB), methodological rigor, possible limitations, and any ethical considerations.

Research Design

Research design is the chosen approach to provide direction for procedures in a research study (Cresswell & Cresswell, 2018, p. 250). Research design is important because it identifies how the research was conducted and it determines the quality of the research procedures. The research design of this study is a nonexperimental qualitative content analysis that uses a qualitative coding technique of secondary data. A qualitative content analysis is a method that identifies themes and patterns in qualitative data (Cresswell & Cresswell, 2018). A qualitative coding technique is a process that organizes data into thematic categories (Cresswell & Cresswell, 2018, p.247). Secondary data are pre-existing datasets created by somebody other than the researcher (Cresswell & Cresswell, 2018). Using this research design will provide many perspectives from app user reviews and will identify areas for improvement and app user's needs. This study will also analyze the top competitors in the market. This research design was chosen because qualitative research is a deductive method to uncover themes that address the research issue (Cresswell & Cresswell, 2018).

Research Setting

Research setting is where the research takes place or is conducted (Cresswell & Cresswell, 2018). The publicly available data was collected from the Apple® App Store® and used to compare app features of potential competitors and to analyze the app reviews of the top three app competitors in the market. The research was conducted online at California State University Bakersfield.

Role of the Researcher and Reflexivity

The role of the researcher is to adopt an unbiased approach to research to ensure their research is not skewed or contains bias. Factors for biases that researchers may have include their values, gender, history, culture, past experiences, and socioeconomic status (Creswell & Creswell, 2018, pp.183 - 184). My background consists of having an undergraduate business degree and experience working with and for small businesses. I also have a personal connection to the business proposal because I created the idea using my family's experiences of diet issues in mind. It is important for the researcher to adopt an unbiased approach because the researcher is the one that will analyze the data and determine how they will conduct and structure their research. To mitigate any potential biases, I will use secondary data that cannot be influenced by my perceptions because it was previously collected and made available to the public. I will use Excel™ to categorize and sort reviews by subject or theme, and the program will count the frequency of the reviews to identify which are the top emerging themes. Using this technique will limit bias because counting the frequency will be a fair way to identify which app reviews are most needed and my personal bias will not interfere with prioritizing which app reviews, I think are most needed.

Sample Frame and Sample Size

A sample frame is an accessible population related to the research that can be sampled (Cresswell & Cresswell, 2018). To establish a sample set, I developed inclusion and exclusion criteria. The sample frame for this study is App Store® data that is related to the research topic. The inclusion criteria included comparing data of apps that are categorized as *medical, health and fitness* apps, and *nutrition* apps. The sample frame further narrowed down the data set by excluding four total apps, two apps that had duplicate listings on the app categories and two apps that were deleted from the App Store® because they no longer comply with the IOS™ App Store® rules. The sample frame consisted of 424 apps from the App Store®.

A sample size is a specific and narrowed down population that represents the entire population sample that you gather your data from (Cresswell & Cresswell, 2018). Since this is qualitative research, the sample size can be determined subjectively by the researcher, rather than having a calculated number for the sample size. Sample size for qualitative study will depend on the number of existing resources available or until a point of saturation is met. The point of saturation is when new data does not provide new information about the data set (Cresswell & Cresswell, 2018, p.250). The sample size for this study is 420 apps. This sample size was determined because I wanted to analyze all apps that have related categories to ensure I did not miss a potential competitor. Additionally, analyzing 420 apps reached the saturation point, where there was not any new information discovered.

Conceptual Model

A conceptual model captures the outline of the process (Cresswell & Cresswell, 2018). I developed a conceptual model to outline the steps of each part of the market research. I have used the construct of strategic management, the competitor analysis, to conduct my market research.

The first step is to survey the market and identify competitors. The conceptual model depicts the sample frame that was used and includes the inclusion and exclusion criteria. It also shows the results of Part One of the market research. The conceptual model visualizes how I categorized the information to identify the emerging themes from Part Two of the market research (Figure 26). Part Two of the market research includes analyzing the app reviews of the top three market competitors that were identified in Part One of the market research. The emerging themes from the prepositions were then used to identify how the review feedback can be implemented into the proposed app to solve app user's needs.

Figure 26

Conceptual Model Competitor Analysis

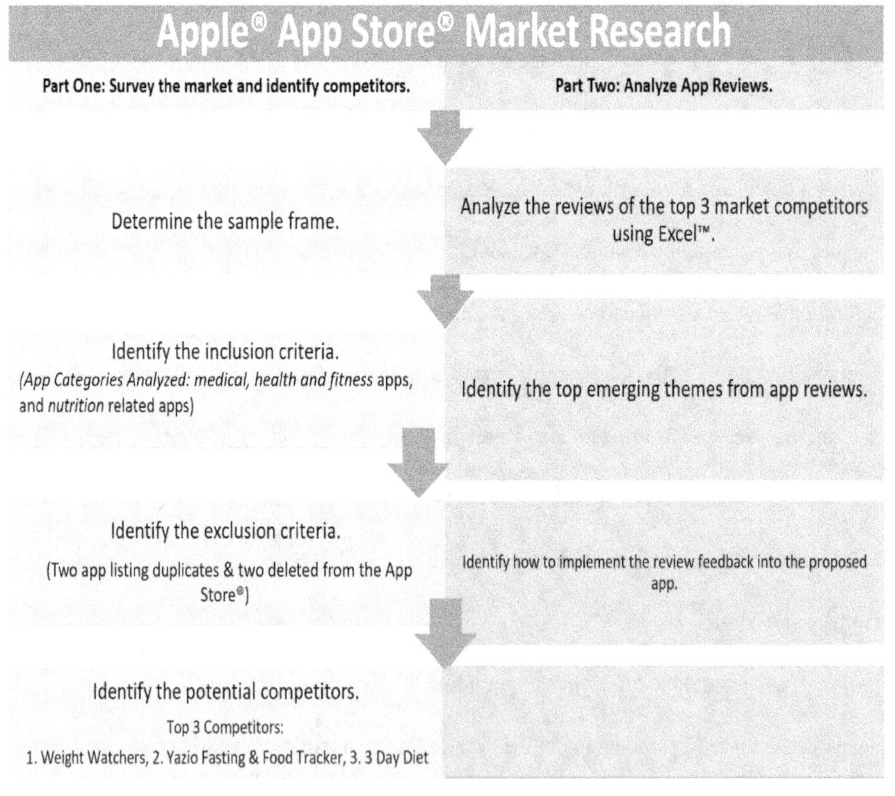

Note. This conceptual model shows how each part of the market research was organized.

Data Collection

A data collection tool is an instrument used to collect data in an organized method (Cresswell & Cresswell, 2018). I developed a data collection tool to use as a checklist to determine if an app was a potential competitor by checking whether the app has similar or shared features as the proposed app. The data collection tool (Appendix H) labeled as *Build My Diet Health App Competitor Analysis Identifying Checklist.* This checklist provides structure to my research by offering a highly organized and reliable method to determine if an app is a potential competitor.

Data Analysis

The market research used a content analysis approach; conducted using a two – step process. I first conducted a competitor analysis of all apps that are *medical, health and fitness* apps, and *nutrition* related apps. I did this by creating a data collection tool checklist that compares potential competitor apps with the app features of my proposed app to identify if they have similar features and can be a competitor. Once I analyzed the apps to the point of saturation, I then counted the frequencies of each category to identify if it is a competitor. The point of saturation is when new data does not provide any new insights (Cresswell & Cresswell, 2018, p.250). The qualitative data collection tool provided a benchmark to limit bias and set a standard criterion of determining whether an app is a competitor. Then I will look at app user reviews of the top three competitors using qualitative coding by counting frequencies of textual data to create a graph. Data analysis was aided by Excel™ and SPSS – R Studio™. This qualitative coding will give insight on app user needs and will categorically reveal trends that need to be improved upon. In summary, the process was as follows: a) collect content, b) sort content by inclusion and exclusion criteria, c) develop and sort content into categories, d) code data, e) count frequencies, f) identify patterns, and g) develop themes. My researching skills were used as the research instrument to determine how to categorize each review, organize the emerging patterns into themes, and applying these themes to the proposed app.

I used the convenience sampling method for my research. The convenience sampling method uses resources and subjects that are chosen based on convenience and availability (Cresswell & Cresswell, 2018, p.150). Examples of convenience sampling in my research are when I chose to use the Apple® App Store®, Excel™, and SPSS RStudio™. Moreover, I used purposeful sampling by establishing inclusion and exclusion criteria for the final sample set. I purposely chose to include the most recent app reviews for the second part of the market research to eliminate personal bias of selecting certain reviews. I only analyzed apps related to my research topic, and I excluded any reviews that directly named somebody in a review, to provide full anonymity.

Methodological Rigor

Methodological rigor is the trustworthiness and accuracy of how the data is displayed. Methodological rigor is important not to misrepresent or misanalyse the data to provide an accurate and consistent interpretation of the data and its protocols (Cresswell & Cresswell, 2018). Since qualitative research is subjective, it is important to ensure that bias does not exist or is limited as much as possible in the study. To establish further credibility of the research, I will establish rigor in my study by creating and including a step-by-step guide of how I conducted my research to facilitate replication of my study.

Internal Validity

Internal validity are the procedures and structure of a study that can influence the outcome of the study, and the researcher's ability to make a correct conclusion of the data (Cresswell & Cresswell, 2018, p. 248). One internal validity threat is instrumentation. Instrumentation is when the data collection tool changes (Cresswell & Cresswell, 2018, p. 171). To limit this threat, I used the same checklist to compare all the apps to determine if they were a competitor or not. Internal validity applies to this study by ensuring that how to guides were included to fully understand how the data was collected.

External Validity

External validity is when researchers can generalize the findings to another situation, setting, or population (Cresswell & Cresswell, 2018, p. 248). This research can be applied to a real – life setting because it uses pre-existing market research data to form a business proposal and develop strategic management strategies. This study has a high external validity because it analyzes data of a real-life market. The types of external validity included in the study are ecological and population validity. Ecological validity is when a research setting or environment is tested to see if it is realistic and can be applied to a real-life setting. Population validity is whether the study uses a large or small sample size (Cresswell & Cresswell, 2018). Examples of ecological validity and population validity in this study are surveying and creating a competitor analysis of a real-life app market. Selection bias is when bias occurs in research (Cresswell & Cresswell, 2018). The selection bias threat was minimized in this study because I selected to analyze apps in all related categories, rather than just doing a competitor analysis of nutrition apps. The generalizability of findings for this study's research design can be used in further research studies because it conducts market research of all apps that are health, medical, fitness, and nutrition related.

Limitations

The limitations of this research project include time restraints and data evolution. Another limitation to my study is access to published apps only. Since I do not have access to unpublished apps, I could not identify and include any future app development threats in my SWOT analysis, because I am unaware of them.

Time restraints were another limitation. More time for research would have included, search engine optimization, or SEO research. This could have been used to uncover which search terms should be included to optimize the search engine to have the app be easier to search for. I chose to only do a competitor analysis of the Apple® App Store® only, since I only had access to the Apple® App Store® and not the Google Play® store.

Institutional Review Board

The IRB is an ethics committee that ensures a proposed research project is ethical and protects the rights of human participants (Cresswell & Cresswell, 2018, p.185). I obtained my training certificate, (Appendix A). Since my study did not include human subject research, the IRB confirmed that this research is out of their review (Appendix B).

Ethical Considerations

Ethical considerations are any issue pertaining to personal disclosure, authenticity, credibility of research, and personal privacy (Cresswell & Cresswell, 2018, p. 88). Respecting app users' confidentiality is an important ethical consideration. Since the App Store® reviews are publicly available data and the users agree to write a public domain review, they forego their privacy rights. However, to further protect privacy of the App Store® reviewers, the reviews will be de-identified to provide full anonymity. The intent of this research is not to cast a negative view of any organizations in this study, but rather create an unbiased factual competitor analysis based on publicly available data.

Chapter 4 - Results

The data was collected from the Apple® App Store® as a two-step market research process. The app reviews were focused on providing insights on app user needs; and categorically revealed trends that need to be improved upon. The first step was to a) conduct a competitor analysis; and the second step was to b) perform qualitative coding on app reviews to discover emerging themes of user's insights. It is crucial to analyze the app reviews and potential market competitors to fully understand the market and user needs; allowing for a well-researched understanding, to develop the business proposal and strategic strategies in chapter five.

Data Collection

Data collection describes the method used to collect the data for analysis (Miles et al., 2020). The data collection for Step One included the creation of a data collection tool that served as the checklist to improve the reliability of the data analysis (Appendix H). I analyzed a broader population of apps by comparing data of apps that are categorized as *medical, health and fitness,* and *nutrition* apps from the Apple® App Store®. The checklist was then used to analyze each app that was identified relevant to the research. Once each checklist was completed, I determined if it was a potential competitor by following inclusion criteria (Appendix G). All apps that were determined to be a competitor were then included in the competitor analysis (Appendix I). The top three competitors were identified to be Weight Watchers™, Yazio™, and 3 Day Diet™ apps.

The data collection for Step Two included the most recent reviews from the Apple® App Store®, and was organized and transferred into an Excel™ workbook. I then determined the top words for each app by counting the frequencies of all the words in the reviews. Once I had counted the frequencies of the most common words, I created a word cloud using a free word cloud generator tool, courtesy of FreeWordCloudGenerator.com. A sentiment analysis was also performed for each review to determine if it was a positive, negative, or neutral review, along with the review's sentiment score. I used an Excel™ add – in to calculate the sentiment score. Lastly, I coded qualitative textual data by identifying brief patterns in each review. I used the Excel™ workbook to organize and code my data into categories and themes.

For both steps of the market research, I researched the copyright permissions to determine if the potential sources could be used in this study. Some potential sources did not allow the copyright permission for this study, so these sources were excluded. I researched the copyright permissions of the Apple® App Store® and the FreeWordCloudGenerator.com, and I found that these sources can be used in the study, as long as I followed their guidelines to properly cite the sources. Build My Diet Health App - A Business Proposal for a Mobile Healthcare App is an independent publication and has not been authorized, sponsored, or otherwise approved by Apple Inc. and are registered trademarks of Apple Inc (required disclaimer).

My initial intent and the anticipated outcome for the data collection of Step One of the market research turned out to be almost the same method of data collection that I planned. Originally, I intended to use the checklist to identify any potential competitors in the market. In the end, I did use the checklist to identify any potential competitors, however, the only limitation was to preserve the dataset by writing down each app name on the checklist, since the dataset was evolving and the App Store® was deleting any apps that did not meet their IOS® update guidelines.

My initial intent for the data collection of Step Two of the market research was to include an existing *How to Guide* for how to conduct market research using SPSS RStudio™. Since the guide was outdated, I could not use SPSS RStudio™. I decided that I was going to use an existing data set of app insights from a third-party organization, so it would be time efficient. I did not use the existing data set due to copyright constraints.

My anticipated outcome for the data collection of Step Two of the market research included data from a source with favorable copyright terms and Excel™ software to store and analyze the data. I decided to use the App Store® to collect data; since it is a direct source of where the reviews originate and tends to improve the rigor of this study.

Data Analysis

In qualitative research, data analysis is the method used to develop categories by coding, count frequencies for priorities, and identify patterns to develop themes using the researcher's objective interpretation (Miles et al., 2020). The original intent for the data analysis for both steps of the market research included creating codebooks and graphs for the qualitative textual data to aid in counting code frequencies and identify any emerging patterns or themes. The only change from my initial plan was to use Excel™ software instead of SPSS RStudio™ to analyze the sentiment reviews and sentiment scores.

Categories were developed for qualitative codes by analyzing each review and identifying similarities and patterns that could be grouped together. The analysis revealed the emerging trends by counting the frequency of codes within a category and showed which patterns were the most prevalent. These emerging trends were organized into a codebook for each of the top three competitors. The top three competitors included Weight Watchers™, Yazio™, and 3 Day Diet™ apps. Each app's codebook was then compared to one another to uncover the common themes they all share. The top emerging themes were identified (Figures 40 & 41). Step – by – step guides for data collection and analysis are appended (Appendix H).

Results

Part One of the Market Research

Part one of the market research included conducting a competitor analysis. The top three competitors were found in the market (Figure 27). All nineteen of the potential competitors in the market were identified and were described in detail (Appendix I). The competitor analysis identifies app features, ratings and reviews score, and languages. The competitor analysis also identifies app categories, awards, in – app purchases, app chart ranking, revenue of the year 2022, and company location. The top three competitors were Weight Watchers™, Yazio ™, and 3 Day Diet™ apps. The Weight Watchers™ app is the leading app in the market, with the Yazio ™ fasting and food tracker app second in the market, and the 3 Day Diet™ app as third in the market. The results of the competitor analysis indicated that the proposed app needs a unique feature for being able to help patients create custom recipes that combine their health condition's dietary restrictions; all with one phone swipe.

Part Two of the Market Research

Part Two of the market research included coding qualitative textual data and creating graphs and figures of the most common words found in each app review of the top three main competitors. The top three competitors were Weight Watchers™, Yazio ™, and 3 Day Diet™ apps. The figures, included word clouds of the most frequent words, and used review sentiment analysis graphs (Figures 28 – Figures 36). All apps had a positive sentiment analysis for the majority of the reviews. The words that were the most frequent in the word clouds of all the apps include *time, good, diet, navigation,* and *app.* The most common words of all the apps are as follows: a) Weight Watchers™: *app, weight,* and *makes* b) Yazio ™: *app, fasting,* and *work*; and c) 3 Day Diet™: *few, app, recommend,* and *simple.*

Figure 27

Comparison of Competitors & Alternative Apps

	Weight Watchers™ (leading app in market)	Yazio Fasting and Food Tracker™	3 Day Diet™
App Features	• NEW integration allows you to connect select CGM (continuous glucose monitor) devices to your WW app to unlock a whole new level of support • Customized food plan and Points Budget • Food, fitness/activity, water, weight, and sleep trackers • Barcode scanner for packaged foods, recipe database, and restaurant database • Progress reports • 24/7 live coach chat • 13,000+ recipes • Blood sugar tracking (with the Weight Watchers Diabetes-Tailored Plan)	• Personal plan to lose weight or build muscles • Calorie table with over 2 million foods • Nutrition tracker and food diary for all meals • Tracks your calories, carbs, proteins and fats • Create meals, add favorites or input new foods • Copy diary entries to other days easily • Built–in barcode scanner for quick searching • Tracks your sports, exercises and activities • Calorie calculator to track your burned calories • Tracks your daily steps walked and be more active • Documents your weight with weight tracker • Assesses your diet and achievements • Syncs with Health App and other fitness apps • Use the Watch App to take control • Great Today widget and 3D touch feature	• At-a-glance meal tracker • Quickly see your day's meals and check them off as you go • Easy-to-read shopping list • Weight loss progress chart • Graphically monitor your weight loss • Personal support • List of approved food substitutions • Customize the diet to your preferences without cheating • Diet Guidelines • Handy reminders to ensure your success over the next three days.
Ratings and Reviews	• 4.8 out of 5	• 4.7 out of 5	• 4.2 out of 5
Languages	• English, Dutch, French, German, Portuguese, Swedish	• English, Czech, Danish, Dutch, Finnish, French, German, Greek, Hungarian, Italian, Japanese, Korean, Norwegian Bokmål, Polish, Portuguese, Russian, Simplified Chinese, Spanish, Swedish, Turkish	• English Only
App Category	• Health and Fitness	• Health and Fitness	• Health and Fitness
In App Purchases	• Yes; and subscription options	• Yes; and subscription options	• $2.99 for app

	• Subscription varies $19.99 - $108.99	• Subscription varies $9.99 - $109.99	
Awards	• #1 Best Diet for Weight Loss 13 years in a row by U.S. News and World Report	• None	• None
App chart of health and fitness apps	• #105	• Not listed	• N/A
2022 Revenue ($USD)	• $36 M Revenue	• $12 M per year	• Not listed
Company Location	• Queens, New York	• Germany	• Not listed

Note. App Store® Data, adapted from Apple®. (2023). *App Store®.* (https://www.apple.com/app-store/).

Figure 28

Weight Watchers[TM] App Frequency Analysis Pareto Charts: Most Common Words

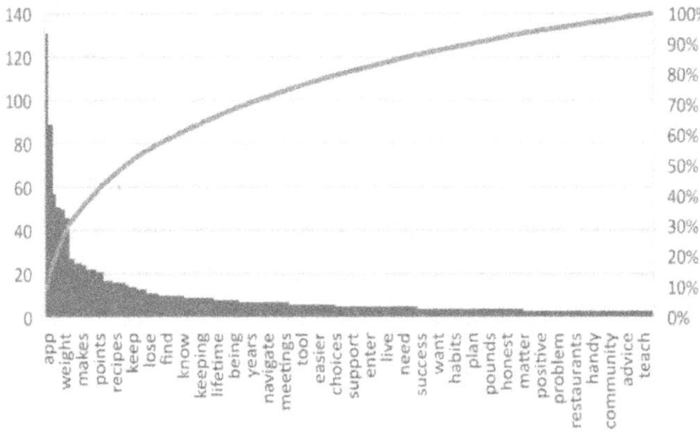

Note. The words that have higher frequencies are the most common words found in the most recent app reviews. I analyzed 178 reviews for the Weight Watchers[TM] app.

App Store® Data, adapted from Apple®. (2023). *App Store®.* (https://www.apple.com/app-store/).

Figure 29

3 Day Diet™ App Frequency Analysis Pareto Charts: Most Common Words

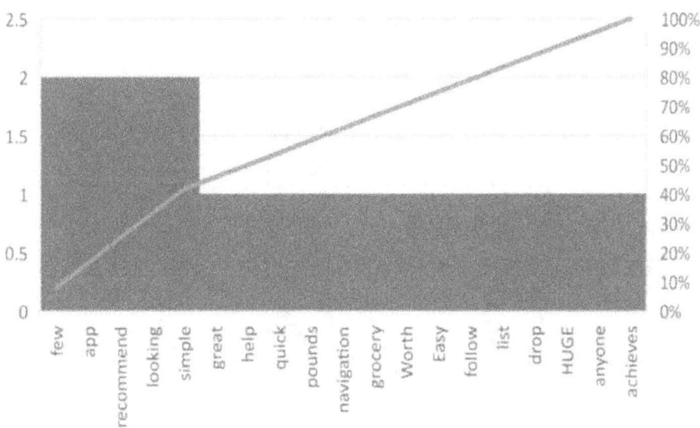

Note. I analyzed two reviews for the 3 Day Diet™ since it only had two reviews listed on the App Store®.

App Store® Data, adapted from Apple®. (2023). *App Store®.* (https://www.apple.com/app-store/).

Figure 30

Yazio Fasting and Food Tracker™ App Frequency Analysis Pareto Charts: Most Common Words

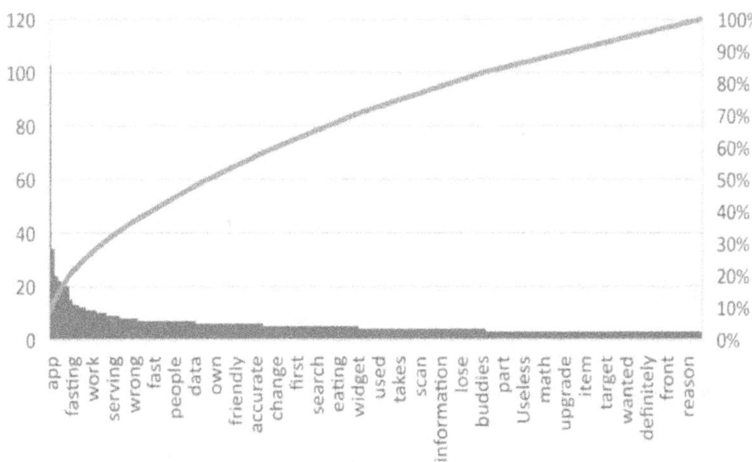

Note. I analyzed 125 reviews for the Yazio Fasting and Food Tracker™ app.

App Store® Data, adapted from Apple®. (2023). *App Store®.* (https://www.apple.com/app-store/).

Figure 31

Yazio[TM] App Frequency Analysis: Distribution of Word Sentiment in App Reviews

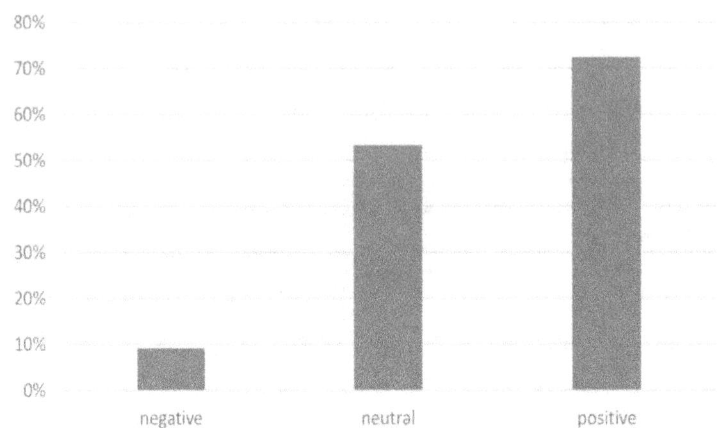

Note. Seventy-two percent of the app reviews were positive for the Yazio[TM] App Frequency Analysis.

App Store® Data, adapted from Apple®. (2023). *App Store®.* (https://www.apple.com/app-store/).

Figure 32

3 Day Diet[TM] App Frequency Analysis: Distribution of Word Sentiment in App Reviews

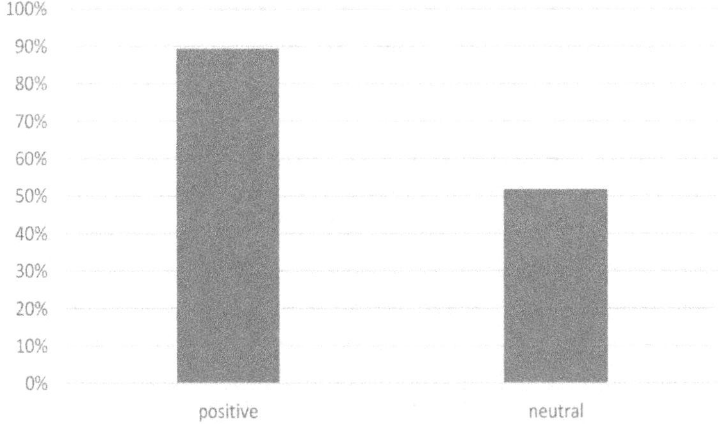

Note. Eighty-nine percent of the app reviews were positive for the 3 Day Diet[TM] App.

App Store® Data, adapted from Apple®. (2023). *App Store®.* (https://www.apple.com/app-store/).

Figure 33

Weight Watchers™ App Frequency Analysis: Distribution of Word Sentiment in App Reviews

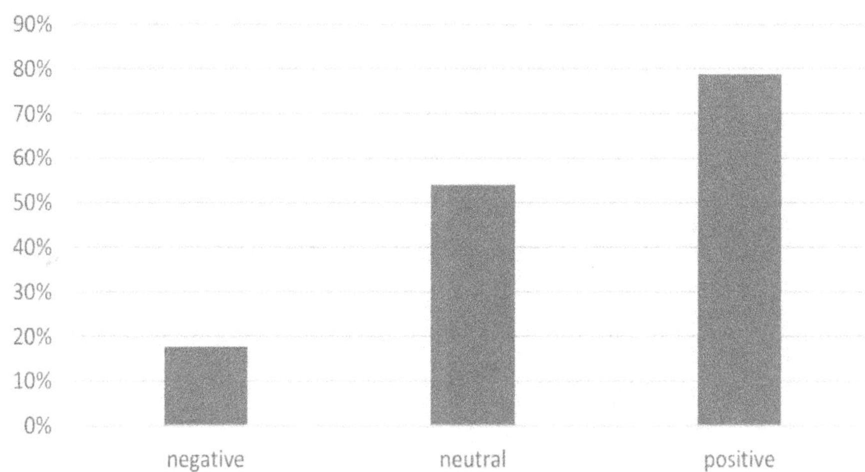

Note. Seventy-nine percent of the app reviews were positive for the Weight Watchers™ App.

App Store® Data, adapted from Apple®. (2023). *App Store®.* (https://www.apple.com/app-store/).

Figure 34

Weight Watchers™ App Frequency Analysis: Word Cloud Where the Frequency of One Word is Reflected By the Size

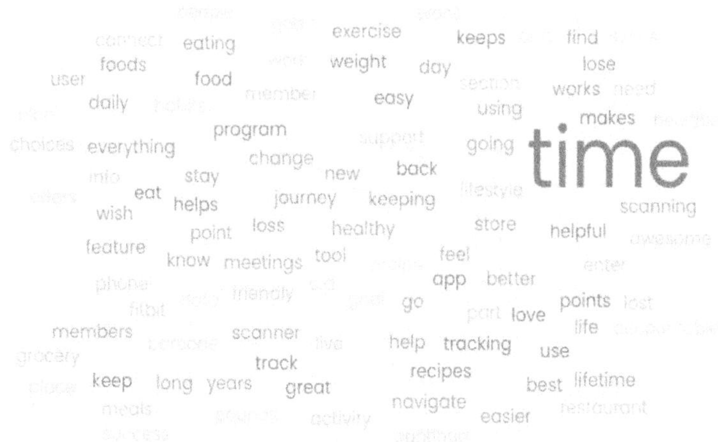

Note. Time is the most frequent word for the Weight Watchers™ App.
App Store® Data, adapted from Apple®. (2023). *App Store®.* (https://www.apple.com/app-store/).

Courtesy of FreeWordCloudGenerator.com

Figure 35

Yazio Fasting and Food Tracker[TM] App Frequency Analysis: Word Cloud Where the Frequency of One Word is Reflected By the Size

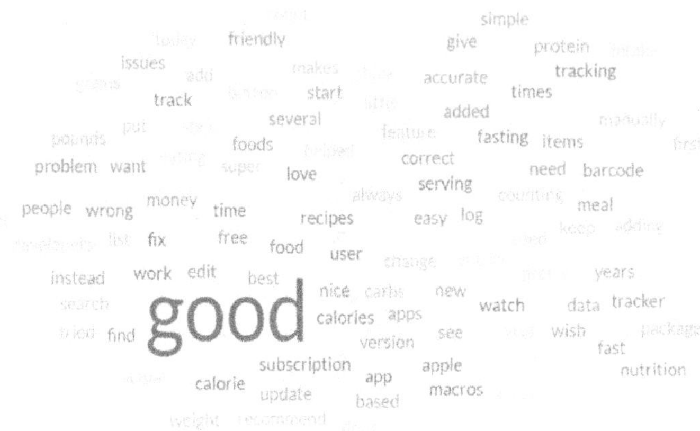

Note. Good is the most frequent word for the Weight Watchers[TM] App.
App Store® Data, adapted from Apple®. (2023). *App Store®.* (https://www.apple.com/app-store/).

Courtesy of FreeWordCloudGenerator.com

Figure 36

3 Day Diet[TM] App Frequency Analysis: Word Cloud Where the Frequency of One Word is Reflected By the Size

Note. Diet, app, feel, navigation, use, different, and *love* were the most frequent words for the 3 Day Diet[TM] App.
App Store® Data, adapted from Apple®. (2023). *App Store®.* (https://www.apple.com/app-store/).

Courtesy of FreeWordCloudGenerator.com

Patterns in the Data Analysis

Parts One and Two of the market research illustrated the frequencies of the codebooks (Figures 37 – Figures 40). The top three categories for each codebook were as follows: a) Weight Watchers[TM]: *love & great app, user friendly & easy to use, and easy tracker for food, scanning, and activities*, b) Yazio [TM]: *needs a better calorie counter & inaccurate nutritional information, buggy and has issues, and love app*; and c) 3 Day Diet[TM]: *simple to use with easy navigation, grocery list feature is nice, and great app.*

Figure 37
Weight Watchers[TM] App Codebook

Category	f	Code
love app / great app	79	a1
easy to use / easy / user friendly	49	a2
easy to track / easy tracking/ track food / easy food tracker / easy food scanner / food tracker / tracks food / track activities	41	a3
Effective / success / helpful / helps	38	a4
accountable	36	a5
lose weight	24	a6
life changer / feel better / better choices	11	a7
Informative / informed	11	a8
Motivating / encouraging	9	a9
Use often	8	a10
points	7	a11
love barcode scanner	6	a12
goals	5	a13
recipes	5	a14
syncs	4	a15
connect to members	3	a16
Fitbit compatible	3	a17
log	3	a18
positive	3	a19

Note. The codebook categories of the Weight Watchers[TM] app show the most frequent to least frequent categories to emphasize which categories are the most prevalent categories. N = 78.

App Store® Data, adapted from Apple®. (2023). *App Store®.* (https://www.apple.com/app-store/).

Figure 38

Yazio[TM] *App Codebook*

Category	f	Code
Needs better calorie counter / wrong calories / wrong serving sizes / inaccurate nutritional information	9	A
Buggy / issues	5	B
love app	5	C
expensive	4	D
Easy to use	4	E
Needs simple interface / needs better integration	4	F
too much personal info	3	G
time consuming	3	H
Too many advertisements	2	I

Note. The Yazio[TM] App Codebook displays categories of improvements for the app. N = 125.

App Store® Data, adapted from Apple®. (2023). *App Store®*. (https://www.apple.com/app-store/).

Figure 39

3 Day Diet[TM] *App Codebook*

Category	f	Code
easy navigation / easy to use / simple	3	a
grocery list feature is nice	2	b
Great app	2	c
feel accomplished / achieve goals	2	d
recommend	1	e
lose weight	1	f

Note. The 3 Day Diet[TM] App Codebook displays favorite features of the app and positive categories. N = 2.

App Store® Data, adapted from Apple®. (2023). *App Store®*. (https://www.apple.com/app-store/).

Figure 40

Summary of Results: Part One and Part Two of the Market Research

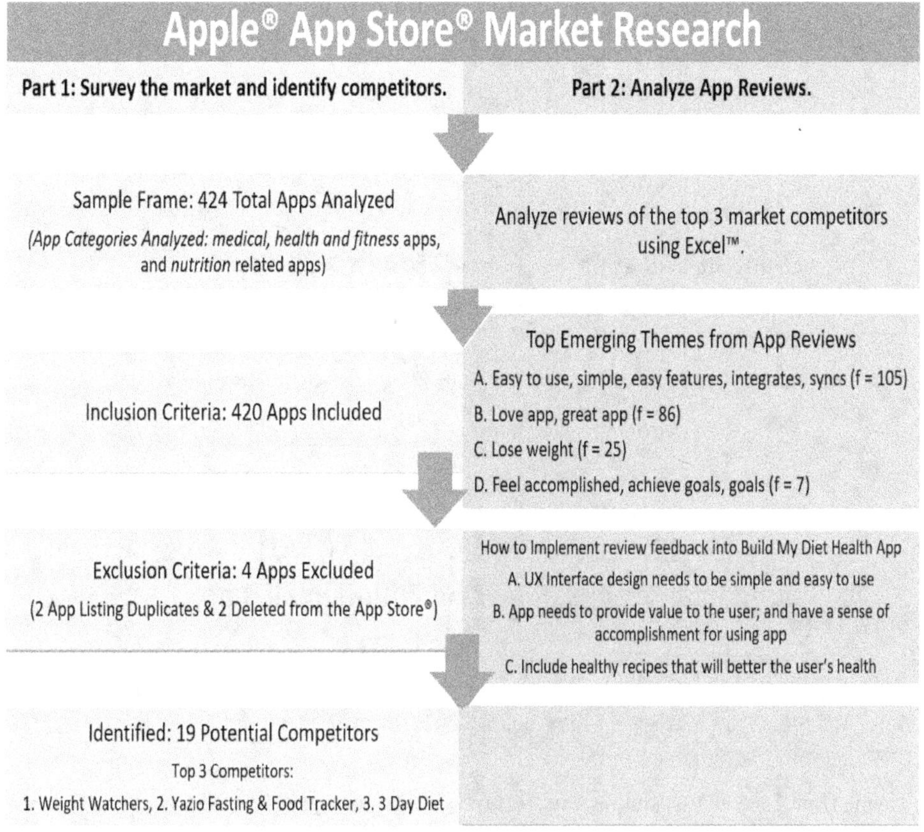

Note. Figure 40 depicts the conceptual model that was developed for this research project. App Store® Data, adapted from Apple®. (2023). *App Store®.* (https://www.apple.com/app-store/).

Themes

The emerging themes from the app reviews were depicted in the data (Figure 41). These themes revealed that the proposed app should be simplistic in design and functionality, should provide health-conscious resources to educate users, and should provide users value and a sense of achievement after using the app. These emerging themes were incorporated into the strategic management strategies for the proposed app in the Chapter 5 business plan.

Figure 41

Emerging Themes from App Reviews

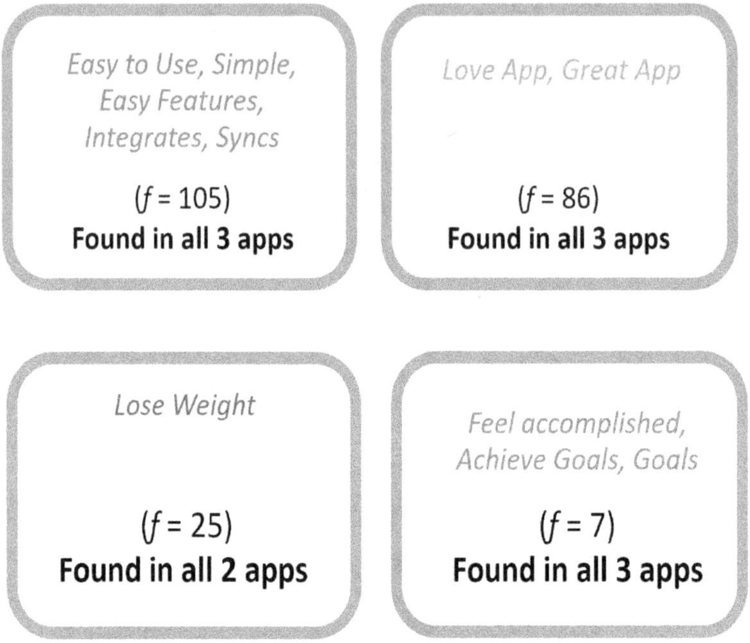

<table>
<tr>
<td>

*Easy to Use, Simple,
Easy Features,
Integrates, Syncs*

$(f = 105)$
Found in all 3 apps

</td>
<td>

Love App, Great App

$(f = 86)$
Found in all 3 apps

</td>
</tr>
<tr>
<td>

Lose Weight

$(f = 25)$
Found in all 2 apps

</td>
<td>

*Feel accomplished,
Achieve Goals, Goals*

$(f = 7)$
Found in all 3 apps

</td>
</tr>
</table>

Note. App Store® Data, adapted from Apple®. (2023). *App Store®.* (https://www.apple.com/app-store/).

Theme One: Easy to use, simple, easy features, integrates, syncs (f = 105)

The first emerging theme indicated that the app needs to be easy to use and functional. This can be applied to the proposed app by ensuring that the UX Interface design will be simple and easy to use. Incorporating a simple interface will reduce the number of errors and will make it easier for users to navigate and save time. Since users will have different technological skills, it is important for the proposed app to be simple for any user to operate and navigate.

Theme Two: Love app, great app (f = 86)

The second emerging theme indicated that the app user's need to love the app and think that it is great. To accomplish this, the proposed app should provide value to the user. An app can provide value to the user by solving an unfulfilled need, and this will lead to increased user engagement. Providing value to the user will increase the user's experience and overall satisfaction. This can be incorporated into the proposed app because it will help patients eat healthier and adhere to their health - constrained diets by providing them with an accessible tool that will create custom recipes based on their diets needs, thereby saving them time.

Theme Three: Lose weight (f = 25)

The third emerging theme indicated that the app needs to help the user lose weight. This can be incorporated into the proposed app by including healthy recipes that will better the user's health. Although weight loss is not the main goal of the proposed app, it is important to include health-conscious resources for users that are interested in improving their overall health.

Theme Four: Feel accomplished, achieve goals, goals (f = 7)

The fourth emerging theme indicated that the app needs to provide a sense of accomplishment by using the app. This emerging theme is similar to the second theme, in that the app needs to provide user satisfaction. This can be applied to the proposed app by incorporating goal setting and monitoring, perhaps on a weekly basis. Additionally, providing the users with the apps valuable services will create user satisfaction and a sense of accomplishment.

Limitations

Although I formed a detailed and thorough structure of the data collection by creating and including the how to guides, there was an unknown and challenging external factor for Step One;

the App Store® *top categories* charts change by the hour in ranking. I solved this issue by

preserving the data order through recording snapshot data collection on a specific day. This

allowed me to preserve the order as much as possible. Since some of the apps mentioned have

been deleted from the App Store® because Apple® is ensuring that each app is up to date with

the new IOS™ App Store® rule compliance, I removed from the study, any apps that I could not

find or were duplicates. There were only two duplicates (Lifesum™ and Weight Watchers™)

and two were deleted from the App Store®. In total, 424 apps were analyzed with four of those

apps being excluded from the competitor analysis and 420 of those apps were included in the

App Store®.

Summary

I used a public domain source, the App Store®, to collect relevant data and conducted a

content analysis on qualitative textual material in the form of app reviews. The analysis provided

insight on app user needs and categorically revealed trends that need to be improved upon. In

summary, the process included: a) data collection, b) sort content by inclusion and exclusion

criteria, c) develop and sort content into categories, d) code data, e) count frequencies, f) identify

patterns, and g) develop themes. I followed the conceptual model (Figure 40), and I used a

checklist (Appendix H) as my data collection tool to provide structure and internal validity

(reliability) for this study. The analysis uncovered that the proposed app in the business plan

needs a unique feature of being able to help people create custom recipes that combine their

health condition's dietary restrictions, all with one phone swipe. The research identified nineteen

potential competitors (Appendix I). The top emerging themes were analyzed and chapter four

described how these themes can be applied to the proposed app (Figure 40).

Chapter 5 – Business Proposal and

Development of Strategic Management Strategies

Chapter five serves as the outcome and end - product of this research. It is a business plan for lowering the massive amount of negative health consequences of poor nutrition by introduction of a new diet management app to the marketplace.

Business Proposal and Strategic Management Strategies

The Problem

With the rising occurrence of chronic and noncommunicable diseases, healthcare interventions need to be developed to help patients navigate their self-management of their conditions. Reducing risk factors for noncommunicable diseases could prevent almost 39 million deaths by 2030, such as implementing a healthy diet, not smoking, exercising regularly, moderating alcohol intake, and reducing exposure to air pollution (Harvard T.H. Chan School of Public Health, 2023). The Build My Diet Health App offers a form of solution to assist patients in adhering to their diets by creating custom recipes they can generate anywhere, anytime. Build My Diet Health App will help patients create recipes that will be tailored to their personal health conditions, and this will save patients time and make it easier for any patient of any educational level to self-manage their health conditions. This app can be impactful because it will make self-management of chronic conditions and diets easier, while addressing the shortage of nutritionists and dietitians in an accessible and cost-effective method.

The current goal of the Build My Diet Health App is to ease the burden of dietary self-management for patients that have chronic conditions. The app will create custom recipes for each patient tailored to their personal health conditions, and patients can have healthier alternatives to their diet adherence.

The long-term goal of the Build My Diet Health App is to create a more efficient lifestyle of self-management by addressing the rising problem of noncommunicable diseases, lack of healthcare resources, and rising healthcare costs. Many patients have been diagnosed with noncommunicable and chronic diseases, but how do these patients manage their chronic conditions? Many are sent home with a printout of what they can eat, and many patients are sent home confused wondering what they can eat with their new chronic disease? The Build My Diet Health App is committed to solve this problem by creating an app that will generate recipes that will be tailored to their personal health conditions and will save patients time and make it easier for any patient to self-manage their health conditions.

Our Solution

Our Mission Statement

The Build My Diet Health App is committed to ease the burden of self-management for patients who face the challenge of managing their noncommunicable and chronic diseases.

Our Vision Statement

Our vision is to create a more efficient and accessible way for any patient, no matter their educational background, to self-manage their health conditions with ease and accuracy. This will create our community members to have better health outcomes and less health complications because they will be likelier to stick to their diet with an intervention that can assist them.

Business Description of Products and Services

Figure 42

Proposed Start Up Screen & Branding

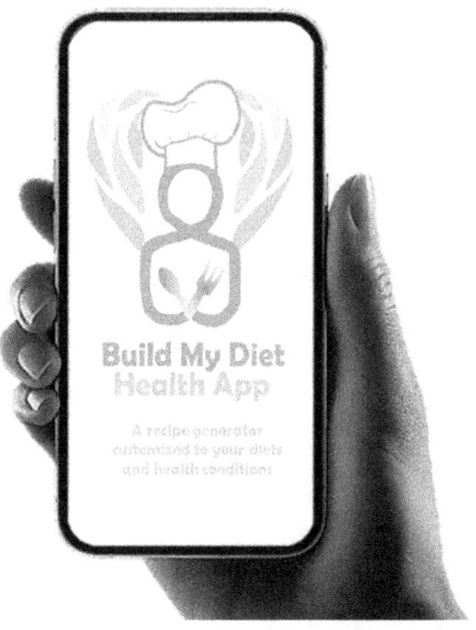

Figure 43

Proposed Profile Screen

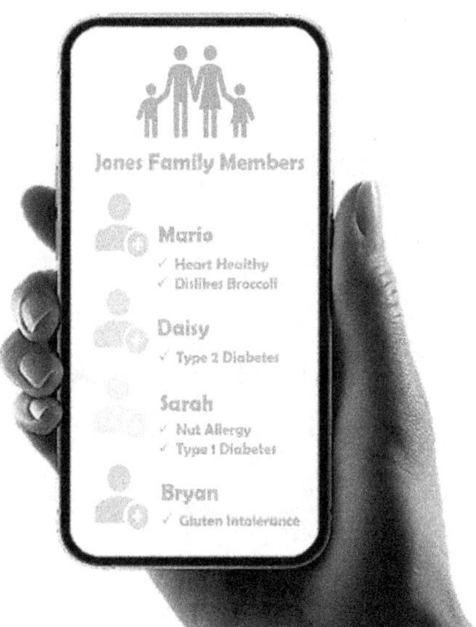

Figure 44

Proposed Home Screen

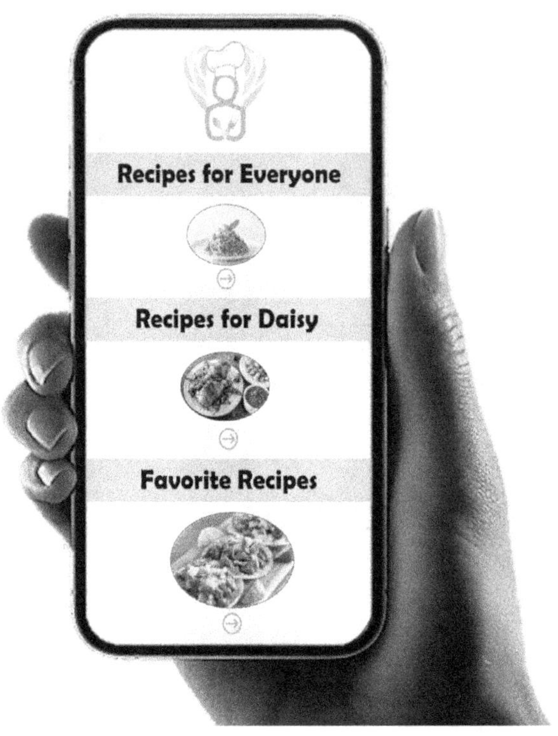

The services include subscription services that will have users pay monthly subscriptions

to use the app to create custom recipes that will align with their health dietary restrictions. There

will be several subscription levels to choose from based on usage and budget. Also, there will be

two different types of subscriptions based on customer type. There will be subscriptions for

business to business of healthcare organizations and business to user subscriptions. Both types of

subscriptions will include different subscription levels based on price point to make our services

meet the different needs of our customers.

Although this is mainly a subscription service-oriented business, the business can also

offer tangible products in the future. One example of a tangible future product line can include to expand the business to offer a meal subscription of meal kits to create customized favorite recipes or create a physical kitchen location to have the staff create the customized meals and deliver it to the customer, so the customer can save time; yet still eat a healthy diet that aligns with their health constraints.

Target Customer

Business to Business, Business to Consumer, or both?

The Build My Diet Health App will be available to both business to business and business to consumer. Business to business is when a business sells its products and services to another company. Business to consumers is when a business directly sells its products or services to the individual customer (Heaslip, 2022). The Build My Diet Health App will implement both business to business and business to consumer. The company can sell its services to individual users (business to consumer) and sell its subscription services to hospitals, hospice organizations, local doctor offices, nutritionists, dietitians, and local public health organizations (business to business). The original goal can be to start off selling business to consumers to spread the word about the proposed app and to fully test out the app in a large setting. Once the app gains traction and works out any technological issues, the company can focus on selling its services business to business of local healthcare organizations. Selling business to business of local healthcare organizations will increase subscription contracts, promote consistent income of sales in large volume, and will help the company establish and grow its brand reputation of being an industry leader.

Business to Business of Healthcare Organizations. These subscriptions will be sold to other healthcare organizations that will allow their patients, members, or employees to access the services. These subscriptions will be yearly subscriptions. A three-month trial can be offered for new healthcare organizations interested in testing our services before contracting with us. Prices will vary by organization depending on contracting terms.

Business to Consumer. These subscriptions will be sold directly from the company to the customer. There are various levels of subscriptions to choose from based on need and budget.

Revenue Model: Types of Subscriptions

Based on the market research from the top competitors, it was found customers are willing to pay on average $20 - $120 for health-related app subscriptions (Appendix I).

Business to Business of Healthcare Organizations.

- **Let's be Chefs! Subscription Level** – Partners receive a 10% discount off their total subscription cost. (Pricing varies depending on how many users an organization will need. The subscription cost is $120 per user per month.)

    - Created for small healthcare organizations.

    - Includes: Unlimited access for up to 500 patients, members, or employees.

- **Foodie Partners Subscription Level** – Partners receive a 15% discount off their total subscription cost. (Pricing varies depending on how many users an organization will need. The subscription cost is $120 per user per month.)

    - Created for midsized healthcare organizations.

    - Includes: Unlimited access for up to 2,500 patients, members, or employees.

- **Epic Cooking Partner Subscription Level** - Partners receive a 20% discount off their total subscription cost. (Pricing varies depending on how many users an organization will need. The subscription cost is $120 per user per month.)

- Created for large healthcare organizations.

- Includes: Unlimited access for more than 2,500 patients, members, or employees.

Business to Consumer.

- **Just a Taste! Subscription Level** - $20 per month

    - Includes: Seven different recipes

- **Chef's Little Helper Subscription Level** - $70 per month

    - Includes: Fourteen different recipes

- **Favorite Foods Unlimited Subscription Level** - $120 per month

    - Includes: An unlimited amount of recipes

Our Location

Since the company is a remote technological company, location is inconsequential. The company's location will be centrally located in Bakersfield, CA. Bakersfield is a good place to start the company because I have grown up in this community, and I am very familiar with the local resources. The main relevance of location is having local network connections and relationships with industry leaders. It is important to be familiar with the area before choosing a company location because each town is unique and there can be unforeseen variables such as culture, local networking ties, resources, talent, and whether a community has enough potential customers to support this new venture. Bakersfield, CA will be a good location for the Build My Diet Health App. There are 77 health care organizations in the greater Bakersfield metro area. These health organizations earn more than $1 billion in revenue each year, and have assets of $1 billion (Cause IQ, 2023, para. 1). Bakersfield has a large healthcare industry to support the

business-to-business model.

Potential Market Size

North America dominated the personalized nutrition and supplements market with a share

of 41.51% in 2022. This is attributable to rising product awareness and increased spending on

health and wellness across the U.S. and Canada (Grand View Research, 2018). The U.S. has a

profitable market size to support the Build My Diet Health App. After initial success in Kern

County, the Build My Diet Health App can be rolled out to the rest of California, the U.S., and the

globe. Please see Appendix B for more charts and figures of the market research of the nutrition

app industry. Figure 45, figure 46, and figure 47 all illustrate two summarized versions of the

market report of the nutrition and dietitian industry, the nutrition and supplements industry, and

the mobile app industry.

Figure 45

Personalized Nutrition And Supplements Market Report Scope

Report Attribute	Details
Market size value in 2023	USD 49.52 billion
Revenue forecast in 2030	USD 131.62 billion
Growth rate	CAGR of 15.0% from 2023 to 2030 to reach USD 131.62 billion by 2030.
Base year for estimation	2022
Historical data	2018 - 2021
Forecast period	2023 - 2030
Quantitative units	Revenue in USD million/billion and CAGR from 2023 to 2030
Report coverage	Revenue forecast, company ranking, competitive landscape, growth factors, and trends
Segments covered	Ingredient, dosage form, distribution channel, age group, region
Regional scope	North America; Europe; Asia Pacific; Latin America; MEA

Country scope	U.S.; Canada; Germany; U.K.; France; Italy; Spain; Denmark; Sweden; Norway; China; Japan; India; South Korea; Australia; Thailand; Brazil; Mexico, Argentina; South Africa; Saudi Arabia, UAE; Kuwait

Note. Personalized Nutrition And Supplements Market Report Scope, adapted from Grand View Research. (2018). *Personalized nutrition and supplements market size, share & trends analysis report by ingredient (vitamins, minerals), by dosage form (liquids, powders), by age group, by distribution channel, and segment forecasts, 2023 - 2030.* (https://www.grandviewresearch.com/industry-analysis/personalized-nutrition-supplements-market-report).

Figure 46

Global App Store® and Google Play® Spending 2021 - 2026

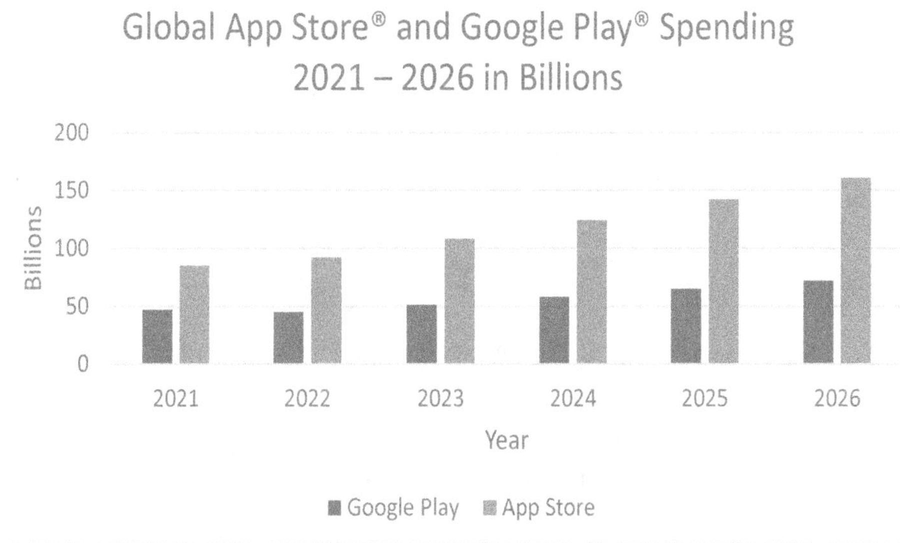

Note. Global App Store® and Google Play® Spending 2021 - 2026, adapted from Velvetech. (2023). *Mobile app development process: Ultimate guide to build an app.* (https://www.velvetech.com/blog/mobile-app-development-process/).

Figure 47

Industry Report

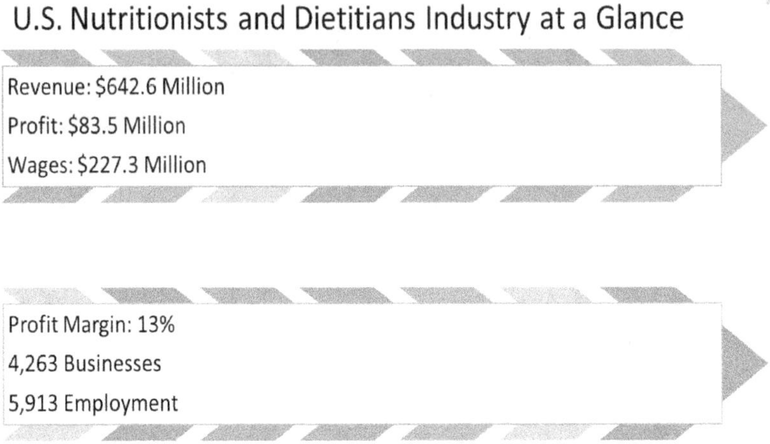

U.S. Nutritionists and Dietitians Industry at a Glance

Revenue: $642.6 Million
Profit: $83.5 Million
Wages: $227.3 Million

Profit Margin: 13%
4,263 Businesses
5,913 Employment

Note. Industry at a Glance, adapted from IBIS World. (2022). *Industry report OD5460:*

Nutritionists and dietitians in the U.S. (https://my-ibisworld-

com.falcon.lib.csub.edu/us/en/industry-specialized/od5460/about).

Financials

The startup financial projections and assumptions are a component of the business

proposal because it includes the projected expenses. It is vital for any organization to calculate a

basic projected budget to determine how much revenue the organization needs to cover its

expenses. Depending on the organization, a lean method can be used by cutting any unnecessary

expenditures that can be substituted for a cheaper alternative that will provide a similar benefit.

The Build My Diet Health App can cut down on cost by using a virtual office space rather than a

physical location in the beginning stages of the organization. Cost can also be reduced by

merging similar job roles together to save on these expenses during the startup phase of the

company. Once the company grows, more employees can be hired, depending on need (Figures

48 & 49). The key to the revenue projections is to utilize contracts and contacts of local

healthcare organizations. Incorporating feedback from local healthcare organizations and having

them be invested in development of the app will help build the exact functionality that the

healthcare organizations want, and the healthcare organizations will be invested in the success of

the app. If the first 6 months or 1 year of initial app rollout go well, the company can ask each

organization to sign a first-option or exclusive contract stipulating that their company has the

first option to create any improvements or successive releases necessary to fully meet the

organization's mobile health app needs. This will serve as a much better way to differentiate than

any particular feature. The software features can also be protected to a limited extent, with trade

secret NDAs for the software logic and copyrights embedded Easter eggs can be hidden within

the actual code, but these by themselves aren't that hard for a competitor to get around; thus, it is

important to have exclusive contracts.

Figure 48

Build My Diet Health App Projected Expenses: Start Up Phase

Category	Item	Projected Cost ($)	Buffer (15%) = $37,989	Alternative Choices Sources
Salaries, Health Insurance, & Benefits	Mobile App Developer Salary	$90,000 per year[1]		Mobile app consultant
	CEO Salary	$90,000 per year[2]		
	~~Nutritionist Salary~~	~~$75,000 per year~~[3]		Work with partnered hospitals & utilize their nutritionist for a short time span as a pilot project.
	Health insurance and benefits for x 2 employees	$13,168 per year[4]		
Marketing Collateral	Website Domain	$45 per year[5]		

	Partnership Collateral Packets	$800 per year[6]		
	Traditional Marketing (ex. Flyers, logo, brochures, vertical banners, business cards, & posters etc.) & Digital Marketing	$7,000 per year[7]		
	Trade Show Tabling Materials	$5,000[8]		
Basic Business Startup Costs	LLC	$95 per year[9]		
	Insurance & Worker's Compensation	$6,852 per year[10]		
	Office Supplies & Equipment (Software, computers, & printers etc.)	$20,000[11]		
	~~Office Lease~~	~~$18,180 per year[12]~~		Use a virtual office space
	P.O. Box	$300 per year[13]		
Travel Expenditures	Conferences, Partnership Meetings, & Trade Shows etc.	$5,000 per year[15]		
Unforeseen Expenditures	Emergency Saving Funds	$15,000[16]		
Total Costs ($)		$253,260	$291,249	

Note. This basic budget includes a 15% buffer in case of inflation or any unforeseen expenses. Alternative choices are also included, and alternative choices are more cost-efficient choices.

[1] Zip Recruiter. (2023). *Mobile applications developer salary in California.* Zip Recruiter. https://www.ziprecruiter.com/Salaries/Mobile-Applications-Developer-Salary--in-California

[2] Zip Recruiter. (2023). *CEO salary in Bakersfield, CA.* Zip Recruiter. https://www.ziprecruiter.com/Salaries/CEO-Salary-in-Bakersfield,CA

[3] Zip Recruiter. (2023). *Registered dietician.* Zip Recruiter. https://www.ziprecruiter.com/g/Highest-Paying-Dietitian-Jobs

[4] Abernathy, T. (2023). *What's the cost of small business health insurance?* Value Penguin. https://www.valuepenguin.com/small-business-health-insurance-

cost#:~:text=The%20average%20small%20business%20owner,the%20company%20and%20the%20worker.

[5 & 6] Shwake, E. (2023). *How much does a domain name cost and why you should buy one?* Wix. https://www.wix.com/blog/how-much-does-a-domain-name-cost

[7] Webfx. (2023). *The cost of marketing: A complex marketing budget breakdown.* Webfx. https://www.webfx.com/digital-marketing/pricing/cost-of-marketing/#:~:text=Companies%20often%20spend%207%2D10,tailored%20to%20its%20Ounique%20needs.

[8] Trade Show Labs. (2023). *Trade Show Costs Statistics.* Trade Show Labs. https://www.tradeshowlabs.com/blog/trade-show-stats#:~:text=The%20average%20cost%20to%20ship,%24500%20to%20%241%2C000%20per%20day.

[9] UpCounsel. (2023). *Understanding California small businesses taxes.* UpCounsel. https://www.upcounsel.com/understanding-california-small-businesses-taxes#:~:text=If%20your%20business%20operates%20as,choose%20to%20form%20in%20California.

[10] Insureon. (2023). *How much does small business insurance cost?* Insureon. https://www.insureon.com/small-business-insurance/cost

[11] Wylie, M. (2020). *How much does it cost to start a business in every industry?* Lending Tree. https://www.lendingtree.com/business/startup-costs-by-industry/

[12] Colliers. (2023). *Office, showroom, and warehouse.* Colliers. https://www.colliers.com/en/properties/officeshowroomwarehouse/usa-3903-patton-way-bakersfield-ca-93308-usa/usa1120613

[13] Capital One. (2023). *How much does a P.O. Box cost?* Capital One. https://www.capitalone.com/learn-grow/life-events/how-to-get-a-po-box/

[14] Collins, H. (2023). *How much does a CPA cost for a small business?* Smart Asset. https://smartasset.com/financial-advisor/how-much-does-a-cpa-cost-for-a-small-business

[15] Hayes, A. (2023). *How much will it cost to hire an accountant to do my taxes?* Investopedia. https://www.investopedia.com/ask/answers/102814/how-much-will-it-cost-hire-accountant-do-my-taxes.asp

The Hartford. (2023). *How much does workers' comp insurance cost?* The Hartford. https://www.thehartford.com/workers-compensation/how-much-does-workers-compensation-cost

[16] Velvetech. (2023). *How much does it cost to make an app in 2023?* Velvetech. https://www.velvetech.com/blog/how-much-mobile-app-cost/

Figure 49

Build My Diet Health App Projected Income: Business to Business Model

	$120.00	Subscription per user per month
x	12 months	1 Year
=	$1,440.00	Subscription per user per year
X	500	Patients
=	$720,000.00	
-	($72,000.00)	10% off exclusive partner discount
=	$648,000.00	
x	8 Healthcare Organizations	10% of total Healthcare Organizations of Bakersfield, CA (77 total healthcare organizations in town)
=	**$5,184,000.00**	**Projected Revenue**
-	($291,249)	Projected Expenses (Figure 45)
-	($460,265.60 per year)	CA Tax Rate of 8.84% of Projected Revenue: $458,265.60 CPA Accountant: $2,000[14]
=	**$4,432,485.40**	**Projected Profit**

Note. This projected income assumes that eight healthcare organizations will purchase a yearly subscription for the *Let's be Chefs! Subscription Level*, which is the subscription level created for the small healthcare organizations of 500 patients. This projected income already calculates in the 10% off discount price for exclusive partners. Assuming 10% of the amount of healthcare organizations in Bakersfield, which is 77 healthcare organizations, purchase a subscription then eight organizations are projected to purchase a subscription (Cause IQ, 2023, para. 1). This only includes the business-to-business model and does not include the business-to-consumer projected revenue.

Differentiation

Competitive Advantage

The competitive advantage is considered both a part of the business proposal and is a

strategic management concept. The competitive advantage for the Build My Diet Health App is

that it has a unique feature that the nineteen potential competitors do not have. The Build My

Diet Health App has a unique feature of differentiation because the app creates custom recipes

for each patient tailored to their personal health conditions, and patients will no longer spend

countless hours researching recipes that adhere to all their diets. The Build My Diet Health App

is focused on a niche to assist patients with their self-management of their dietary constraints

caused by chronic conditions. Some potential competitors contain recipes for chronic conditions;

but they do not combine several diets together to adhere to a patient's full need of combining all

their dietary restrictions into one recipe.

Having a unique feature that has a strong value proposition is an example of the

differentiation strategy because the Build My Diet Health App will stand out against the

competitors (Founder Jar, 2022, para. 6). There are nineteen similar potential competitors, but

these apps are more focused on weight loss, calorie counting, or providing a food weight loss

journal.

The second competitive advantage will be incorporating feedback from local healthcare

organizations and having them be invested in the development of the app, developing the app to

the exact functionality that the healthcare organizations want. If the first 6 months or 1 year of

initial app rollout go well, the company can ask each organization to sign a first-option or

exclusive contract stipulating that their company has the *first option* to create any improvements

or successive releases necessary to fully meet the organization's mobile health app needs. This will serve as a much better way to differentiate than any particular feature. The software features can only be protected to a limited extent, and incorporating exclusive contracts into the strategy of differentiation will set the company apart from the competitors.

The Build My Diet Health App will develop the app in partnership with the local healthcare organizations to lock in the organizations with first – option contracts. Developing the app in partnership with the local healthcare organizations and using the specific chronic conditions, recipes, and dietary restrictions of the healthcare organizations specific patient bases and then doing a good job of delivering on this functionality for the year immediately following launch, will give the Build My Diet Health App a huge advantage against the competitors. The Build My Diet Health App will have a huge advantage in copying competitors' features and building them into the app, which is already customized for your customers' patient bases, compared to the competitors, who would have to *start from scratch,* becoming familiar with the healthcare organizations unique patient bases, to do similar customization.

Market Research: Competitor Analysis

The competitor analysis compares app features, ratings and reviews score, and languages. The competitor analysis also identifies app categories, awards, in – app purchases, app chart ranking, revenue of the year 2022, and company location of each app (Figure 50). Creating this comparison will highlight the strengths, weaknesses, and areas of opportunity in the market. A competitor analysis is found in both strategic management and the business proposal (Ginter et al., 2018). The competitor analysis is found in the business proposal as the market research. The competitor analysis is a part of strategic management by using offensive and defensive strategies of identifying strengths and weaknesses of each app. Offensive strategies are ways for a company to be flexible and defensive strategies are ways for a company to focus on how to

control the market and maintain their market position (Ginter et al., 2018 & Founder Jar, 2022).

Figure 50

Build My Diet Health App Competitor Analysis: A Comparison of Competitors & Alternative Apps

	Weight Watchers™ (leading app in market)	Yazio Fasting and Food Tracker™	3 Day Diet™
App Features	• NEW integration allows you to connect select CGM (continuous glucose monitor) devices to your WW app to unlock a whole new level of support. • Customized food plan and Points Budget • Food, fitness/activity, water, weight, and sleep trackers • Barcode scanner for packaged foods, recipe database, and restaurant database • Progress reports • 24/7 live coach chat • 13,000+ recipes	• Personal plan to lose weight or build muscles. • Calorie table with over 2 million foods • Nutrition tracker and food diary for all meals • Tracks your calories, carbs, proteins, and fats. • Create meals, add favorites, or input new foods. • Copy diary entries to other days easily • Built–in barcode scanner for quick searching. • Track your sports, exercises, and activities.	• At-a-glance meal tracker • Quickly see your day's meals and check them off as you go. • Easy-to-read shopping list • Weight loss progress chart • Graphically monitor your weight loss • Personal support • List of approved food substitutions • Customize the diet to your preferences without cheating. • Diet Guidelines

	• Blood sugar tracking (with the Weight Watchers Diabetes-Tailored Plan)	• Calorie calculator to track your burned calories. • Tracks your daily steps walked and be more active. • Documents your weight with a weight tracker. • Assesses your diet and achievements. • Syncs with Health App and other fitness apps • Use the Watch App to take control. • Great Today widget and 3D touch feature	• Handy reminders to ensure your success over the next three days.
Ratings and Reviews	•4.8 out of 5	•4.7 out of 5	•4.2 out of 5
Languages	•English, Dutch, French, German, Portuguese, Swedish	•English, Czech, Danish, Dutch, Finnish, French, German, Greek, Hungarian, Italian, Japanese, Korean, Norwegian Bokmål,	•English Only

		Polish, Portuguese, Russian, Simplified Chinese, Spanish, Swedish, Turkish	
App Category	•Health and Fitness	•Health and Fitness	•Health and Fitness
In App Purchases	•Yes, and subscription options. •Subscription varies $19.99 - $108.99	•Yes, and subscription options. •Subscription varies $9.99 - $109.99	•$2.99 for app
Awards	•#1 Best Diet for Weight Loss 13 years in a row by U.S. News and World Report	•None	•None
App chart of health and fitness apps	•#105	•Not listed	•N/A
2022 Revenue ($USD)	•$36 M Revenue	•$12 M per year	•Not listed
Company Location	•Queens, New York	•Germany	•Not listed

Note. App Store® Data, adapted from Apple®. (2023). *App Store®.* (https://www.apple.com/app-store/).

Market Research: SWOT Analysis

The SWOT analysis is both a component of the business proposal and it is a concept of strategic management because it is a tool used in strategic management planning and is found in a business proposal during the market research. Analyzing the Build My Diet Health App using a SWOT analysis, there are more positive strengths and opportunities than weaknesses and threats (Figure 51).

Figure 51

Build My Diet Health App SWOT Analysis

	Strengths	**Weaknesses**
Internal	• Target Market: Using exclusive contracts with healthcare organizations will serve as a strong strategy of differentiation that will be difficult for competitors to replicate. • Value Proposition: The app has a unique feature that the competitors do not have. The app will increase efficiency for healthcare organizations and solves a problem for users and healthcare organizations. • Business Model: Virtual location will reduce business expenses.	• Competitive Ecosystem: The market has a medium level of competition with 19 potential competitors.
	Opportunities	**Threats**
External	• Business Model: Virtual location can expand out the business to a statewide, nationwide, and global wide level. • Since it is a B2B & B2C business model, there are a lot of sales opportunities. • Target Market: Healthcare organizations & direct consumers; provides a wider sales base	• Competitive Ecosystem: Other apps are more well known and have well established brand awareness. • Competitive Ecosystem: Other apps may want to add this feature and try to replicate it.

Note. This SWOT analysis displays the internal and external factors of the Build My Diet Health App.

Industry Analysis

An industry analysis is found in both strategic management and the business proposal. According to the market research that was found in chapters one and three, there is a large enough market demand and industry growth for this to be a successful business (Appendix C).

For my industry analysis, I have chosen to conduct a competitor analysis of the apps in the related markets of the 2023 *top categories of health and fitness* and *medical app categories* from the Apple® App Store®. This analyzed the *top free, top paid*, and *best nutrition tracking app categories*. All these categories are related to the research topic at hand; and provide a thorough analysis of any potential competing apps (Appendix I). With a medium competition environment and a high demand for services, this app during its first years of development will have a monopoly in its industry; since the proposed app has a unique feature that the rest do not and exclusive contracts and partnerships with local healthcare organizations will be formed that will be extremely difficult for competitors to replicate (Appendix I).

Operational Plan

The operational plan is a basic component of the business proposal because it outlines the basic operations that are needed to run the organization. The operational plan of the Build My Diet Health App will need to include a mobile app developer, a help desk team that will help users, a nutritionist, and a CEO. As the company grows, an executive assistant, operations manager, marketing manager, an accountant, and an HR manager will need to be hired (Figure 52). Below is an operational plan of how each stage gate will support the hiring of new employees by each phase of the company. This will achieve specific proof-of-concept rollout goals and will bring in progressive amounts of revenue at each stage. The additional revenue at each stage can then be leveraged to acquire more capital and invest in the hiring described (Figure 52). According to the projected income of each stage gate phase, the hiring of new employees will be feasible. The revenue of each stage gate can sustain the hiring of ten employees with salaries of $100,000 each with health insurance and benefits of $6,584 per employee, for a total cost of $1,065,840 for hiring up to the full expansion phase of ten total employees. This will still leave the company with profitable margins.

Stage Gates of Each Business Phase:

- ***Start Up Phase***: 8 local healthcare organizations located in Bakersfield x $648,000 cost of partnership subscription per year for 500 patients of a healthcare organization = ***$5,184,000 revenue***

- ***Growth Phase:*** 8 Bakersfield healthcare organizations + 4 additional healthcare organizations in CA (statewide) x $648,000 cost of partnership subscription per year for 500 patients of a healthcare organization = ***$7,776,000 revenue***

- ***Expansion Phase:*** 8 Bakersfield healthcare organizations + 4 additional healthcare organizations in CA (statewide) + 4 national healthcare organizations x $648,000 cost of partnership subscription per year for 500 patients of a healthcare organization = ***$10,368,000 Revenue***

Figure 52

Build My Diet Health App Organizational Chart

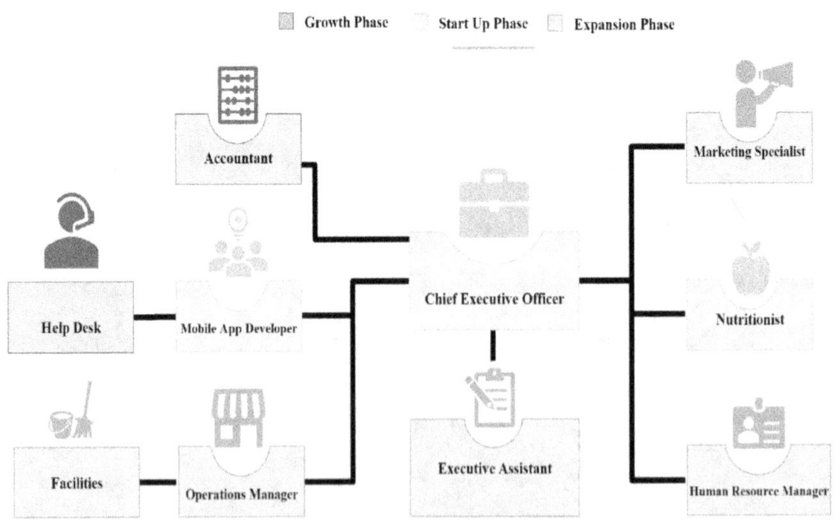

Note. This chart shows the needed talent acquisition for the startup and growth phase; and displays how the organization will change in organization as it develops.

Next Steps to Ensure Our Existence

Overall, this study suggested the Build My Diet Healthcare App can be a successful and profitable business idea because it has a unique feature, it solves a market needed problem, and it creates value for the patients. These steps are important to follow to ensure the Build My Diet Health App company will ensure its existence and will grow from an idea into a company. These steps are strategic management concepts because they include the short- and long-term goals that the company would like to achieve.

Step 1: Define requirements in partnership with local healthcare organizations.

- Provide feedback on what your organizational needs consist of.
- Commit to a common mission.
- Contribute to the partnership with organizational resources, such as assigning a temporary nutritionist to help develop the app etc.
- Be a good steward of partnership resources and keep in constant communication with regular attendance of meetings.

Resources You Have Currently - Resource Requirement:

- Network connections of myself, Dr. Woods, Dr. Pallitto, & other community leaders
- Skillsets: Business and marketing experience
- Cash on Hand: $5,000
- Borrowing Capacity: $22,500 (30% of $75,000 income)
- Grant Funding Target: We will make investments of up to $3,000,000 over the life of a company, with the original investment likely between $50,000 and $250,000 for companies at the seed stage and up to $1,000,000 for growth stage (California Health Care Foundation Innovation Fund for Entrepreneurs, 2023).

Resource You Will Need in the Future - Resource Requirement:

- 8 Partnerships with local healthcare organizations that are willing to provide feedback on their organization needs.

Step 2: Weave AI consideration into the development, testing, and rollout phases of the app.

Artificial intelligence will be considered to use iteratively throughout the process, as various features and code will be developed. Using artificial intelligence will be a lean method, because it will quickly and efficiently assist the app developer to build the app. The Build My Diet Health App can also incorporate artificial intelligence into the app to generate recipes custom to the needs of the patients. This can potentially reduce wait times, and patients will no longer have to wait until their next appointment to receive newly made recipes for the patient. Also, the recipes can be reviewed by a nutritionist to ensure that all recipes align with the patient's diets to reduce any liabilities. Considering how artificial intelligence can be incorporated into the app will be an important next step because this app can be a time efficient tool that will help nutritionists, healthcare organizations, and patients improve their health outcomes and address this shortage of healthcare professionals.

Resource You Will Need in the Future - Resource Requirement:

- 1 artificial intelligence software program

Step 3: Develop the app and follow the business proposal.

Developing the app and following the business proposal will be the next step. A software developer with technical knowledge and skills will need to be hired or be made into a business partner to develop the app. Following the business proposal and putting the plan into action will turn this concept into a reality.

Resource You Will Need in the Future - Resource Requirements:

- 1 mobile app developer

- Office Supplies and equipment for three employees

Step 4: Conduct a pilot trial of the app to test it out and improve the app based on the pilot trial results.

After the app is developed, it is imperative to test it out before releasing it for public use. It is important to have a quality improvement process in place, and this can be a method to use to test the quality and improve upon what is needed. It is important to test it out first to ensure the app is accurate and efficient to use without any issues. The best way to do this is to test it out using a pilot trial. A pilot trial will be a cost-effective method to test out any issues because it will simulate a short-term study to see how the app will function in a real-life setting. It is important to collect the feedback of the pilot test trial users and to improve the app based on these results. It is vital that the final app version will have minimum errors because users will not trust the app and the reputation of the app can be jeopardized if it is known as an app that does not work well or has lots of issues.

Resource You Will Need in the Future - Resource Requirements:

- 8 Partnerships with local healthcare organizations that are willing to do a pilot trial of the app to provide feedback on their organization needs and provide us with app performance feedback.

Step 5: Release the app to progressively larger pilot populations; expand languages, app features, and accessibility on a needed basis.

Releasing the app for public use will allow for greater feedback from users on the app's performance. This can uncover trends of needed app features or will lead to feedback that can improve upon the app's performance. This can lead to the discovery of new app features that are needed and can lead to greater accessibility. Also, the app can expand its language base on a needed basis, to serve a wider demographic. Quality improvement is an iterative process; and incorporating user feedback is vital to understand the patient's needs and problems. Expanding languages in mobile health technologies is important in achieving health equity and increasing accessibility for all populations. The Build My Diet Health App will be a popular tool in rural areas because these locations have the most need for a health intervention tool such as this one. Typically, rural areas are communities that have diverse languages and uncovering which languages are most needed and incorporating them into the app will allow greater accessibility and serve a wider demographic of patients.

Resource You Will Need in the Future - Resource Requirements:

- 8 Partnerships with statewide and nationwide healthcare organizations that are willing to do a pilot trial of the app to provide feedback on their organization needs and provide app performance feedback.

- Expand our staff levels of the Build My Diet Health App & hire 7 new additional employees to the team, for a total of 10 employees.

- Find a physical office space and purchase more office equipment and supplies for the 7 new employees.